MEDICAL ENGLISH USAGE AND ABUSAGE

By Edith Schwager

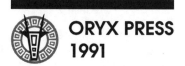
ORYX PRESS
1991

The rare Arabian Oryx is believed to have inspired the myth of the unicorn. This desert antelope became virtually extinct in the early 1960s. At that time several groups of international conservationists arranged to have 9 animals sent to the Phoenix Zoo to be the nucleus of a captive breeding herd. Today the Oryx population is nearly 800, and over 400 have been returned to reserves in the Middle East.

Copyright © 1991 by Edith Schwager
Published by The Oryx Press
4041 North Central at Indian School Road
Phoenix, Arizona 85012-3397

Published simultaneously in Canada

Printed and Bound in the United States of America

∞ The paper used in this publication meets the minimum requirements of American National Standard for Information Science—Permanence of Paper for Printed Library Materials, ANSI Z39.48, 1984.

Library of Congress Cataloging-in-Publication Data

Schwager, Edith.
  Medical English usage and abusage / by Edith Schwager.
    p. cm.
  Includes bibliographical references (p. 189).
  Includes index.
  ISBN 0-89774-590-6
  1. Medical writing. 2. English language—Medical English.
I. Title.
R119.S38   1991   90-7644
808'.06661—dc20   Rev. CIP

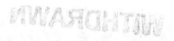

To the memory of my father, Michael, to Karen,
my daughter, for her unwavering encouragement
and beauty of spirit, and to Michael, my son, for
his inspiration and perspiration

Contents

Tower of Babel curse ○ English as world language ○ Illiteracy of
the educated and miseducated ○ Preserving the language

Homophony ○ Egregious errors in cold print ○ Freudian slips
and misquotation ○ Miscomprehension ○ Mixed metaphors ○
Typographic errors ○ Scrambled medical knowledge ○
Proofreading

Abstracts ○ Agonist, antagonist ○ Apgar score ○ AZT, Retrovir,
and AIDS ○ Bacteria ○ Caduceus ○ Capitalization in headings ○
Cesarean, Caesarean, cesarean, or caesarean? ○ Cf. ○ Column
heads in tables ○ Consistency of terms ○ Cross and hyphens ○
Dana-Farber Cancer Institute ○ Describing techniques and
methods ○ Decimals and less than one ○ Decimals and tables ○
Decimals that can kill ○ D.M.D. ○ Double-spacing of
manuscripts ○ Endemic, epidemic, pandemic, epizootic ○
Eponyms ○ Errors in lists of references ○ Hyphens in titles ○
ISBN ○ Justified lines in manuscripts ○ Leonardo da Vinci ○
Liter ○ Logotype ○ Morbidity, mortality rates ○ Numbers and
consistency ○ Oxygen ○ Personal communications ○ pH value ○
Pixel ○ Points and periods ○ Proprietary and nonproprietary

names ○ q.v ○ Smithsonian Institution ○ Titles of journals and books ○ Trademarked names ○ Vestigial tails ○ Virgule and per ○ von ○ YAG ○ ZIP code

Abstractions and plurals ○ Active vs. passive voice ○ And or or ○ As best as ○ As good as ○ Between the cracks ○ Blame on ○ Compare to, with ○ Dangling modifiers ○ Different from, different than ○ Disagreement in number of verb ○ Dissimilar ○ Drug, dragged ○ Ensure, insure ○ Equally as ○ Fewer, less ○ Fit, fitted ○ Fly ○ I, we ○ If, whether ○ In, into ○ Lay, lie ○ Ligatures ○ One who ○ Other ○ Parallelism ○ Pit, pitted ○ Preposition at end of sentence ○ Proved, proven ○ Since, because ○ Singular or plural verb? ○ Split infinitives ○ Subjunctive ○ That, which ○ Under way ○ Who, whom

Administer ○ Aggravate ○ Authored ○ Center around ○ Compendium ○ Fewer, less ○ Fractions and parts thereof ○ Incomparables ○ Minimize, minimum ○ Relations, relationships ○ Tandem ○ Vicious circle

Apostrophes: Elision ○ Possessives of nouns ○ Possessive "of" understood ○ **Commas:** Apposition ○ Commas between adjectives ○ Dates and commas ○ Senior, Junior, and the Third ○ Serial comma ○ **Ellipses** ○ **Hyphens:** Adverbs modifying adjectives ○ Chemical substances as modifiers ○ Clarifiers ○ Compound verbs ○ Foreign phrases ○ In vitro, in vivo ○ Medical conditions and entities ○ Non-, co-, -less, and other affixes ○ Nouns combined with adjectives ○ Nouns linked to nouns ○ Prefixes and proper nouns ○ Re- words ○ Spelled-out words and numerals ○ Unhealthful hyphens ○ The word processor and hyphenation ○ Year-long ○ **Parentheses** ○ **Periods** ○ **Quotation Marks**

And/or ○ In another vein ○ In any case ○ Like, such as ○ Operation ○ Patency, patent ○ Significant

Foreword

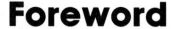

I cannot imagine an area of human endeavor in which precise communication is more important or in which its lack can have more devastating consequences than medicine. Many of the examples in this excellent work are humorous; I know of others that are fatal. "Am I clearly saying what I mean?" must always be uppermost in the mind of every writer on medical topics.

All of us can learn from Edith Schwager: physicians and other health professionals who note observations and issue written instructions, scientists who record laboratory findings and write the results for publication, journalists who interpret those same results for the reading public, and even experienced editors—those indispensable watchdogs who attempt to keep the rest of us from making fools of ourselves in print.

I had to read no further than the title of this work to learn something. "Abusage," although not in my desk dictionary, has one meaning in *Webster's Third*: "Improper or incorrect use of language: bad usage." Exactly the right word.

Medical English Usage and Abusage is both a source of guidance, to be consulted when occasion demands, and a source of pleasure, engagingly written, to be dipped into for inspiration.

Donald A. B. Lindberg, M.D.
Director, National Library of Medicine

Preface

The number of high school graduates going on to colleges and universities is steadily increasing, but the amount of pitiable writing that you and I see proves that postgraduate help is essential.

Almost everyone in business or the professions is called on at some time or another to write, whether it's a memorandum or a monograph, a letter or a laboratory record, an article or an advertisement. Too frequently what they produce would make their former teachers disavow them.

Many motives impelled me to write this book.

What orchestra conductor would be satisfied to hear a C in a Beethoven composition when the score shows a D? What arithmetic teacher would sit still for 12 as the sum of 8 and 5? Yet some teachers, writers, and editors settle too easily for the word or phrase that is almost right. Mark Twain wrote, "The difference between the right word and the nearly right word is the same as that between lightning and the lightning bug."

The rules of usage are like traffic laws—easy to obey if you are familiar with them. Incredible though it may seem, most traffic rules are there for good reason. All but the most airheaded, reckless, and ignorant take them seriously. Those who disobey do so at their peril.

People who consider it practical, daring, clever, chic, or innovative to disobey usage rules risk being misunderstood—a fate most painful to us professionals and therefore to be avoided.

Usage changes. That's fortunate—and inevitable. The archaic, obsolete, or quaint should be replaced. But chaos should not reign. Usage is whatever the good speakers, writers, and editors in America say it is at any given moment. Note the "good." It excludes people who never took advantage of compulsory education, those who never read, those who consider themselves above the law (of usage), and those who couldn't care less.

In his preface, "A Word to the Whys," of *Miss Thistlebottom's Hobgoblins*, Theodore Bernstein wrote, "What we require is neither a language that is cramped nor a language gone wild."

Dictionaries and usage books exist not to fulfill some deep-seated prissiness on the part of their writers; they are written to resolve disputes without acrimony. They save the valuable time of writers, editors, speakers, and others interested in expressing themselves intelligently, clearly, economically, and stylishly.

This book on medical English usage and abusage in the American manner is for anyone working in medicine or pharmaceuticals or the allied health fields: writers, editors, journalists, laboratory technicians, psychologists, hospital administrators, advertising, public relations, and audiovisual workers, teachers, translators, researchers, physicians, nurses, and medical students.

Much of the material in this book is influenced by the bright, receptive students who have attended my seminars and workshops on English and medical English usage over the past 25 years, particularly those conducted under the auspices of the American Medical Writers Association.

In medical writing, there is no danger in being too precise—only in being imprecise.

This is a book on usage, not grammar. The mistakes I discuss are mainly the result of:

- poor training or education, whether of the formal or unstructured kind;
- the wrong word order in a sentence;
- miscomprehension of everyday or abstruse, technical terms used in speech or writing;
- the lack of handy reference material;
- the profusion of homophones and homographs in the English language;
- carelessness stemming from complaisance, complacency, or the pressure of deadlines;
- and the all-too-human desire to appear learned.

The *United Nations Statistical Yearbook: 1983-84*, stated that 16 percent of the primary school students in the world, and 77 percent of the secondary school students, are studying English. In the Soviet Union, more than 50 percent of the high school students study English. More than 437 million people throughout the world speak English.

Several factors weigh heavily in favor of modern-day American English as the world language, although more people speak other principal languages. (Mandarin and its variants are spoken by more than 844 million people.) It is not a highly inflected language. Its spare inflection, especially in comparison with other predominant world languages, is probably one compelling reason for its becoming the world language, despite its illogical, difficult, and inconsistent spelling. The political and economic power of the United States and the democratic example it sets also contribute greatly to its success.

Our medium—the English language—is our message to the world.

Credibility, hard-earned, is what writers have to offer. It is the *sine qua non.* To paraphrase a James M. Barrie character (who was talking about charm), if you have credibility, you hardly need to have anything else; if you don't have it, it doesn't much matter what else you have.

Editors and anyone who writes, whether professional or amateur, may find my book useful as a practical, sometimes irreverent guide to medical English usage, American style.

Samuel Johnson's aphorism is as apt now as when he wrote it: "A man will turn over half a library to make one book." I have turned over all of my library.

When Billie Dawn, in the play *Born Yesterday*, is challenged on her use of a word, she and her tormentor consult the dictionary. She's wrong. "Well," she says defiantly, in her endearingly high-pitched but wistful voice, "that's one man's opinion."

This book is one woman's opinion.

Acknowledgments

Can an author acknowledge all the individuals and organizations that helped make a book without offending some because they are not included and others because they are?

I'll try.

I thank Michael J. Schwager, a writer and my favorite editor. Without him—my gifted son, my introducer to the world of word processing—this book would not, quite literally, have been possible, at least not by the deadline.

I give special thanks to the members and staff of the American Medical Writers Association, from whom I have learned so much over the past 26 years and to whom I owe so much for their faith and friendship. The publisher frowns on printing 3,300 names.

I give special thanks also to the readers of my "Dear Edie" column in the *AMWA Journal* and its predecessor, *Medical Communications*. Their queries have enriched my life by challenging my research and writing skills and thereby providing countless hours of enjoyment.

My heartfelt thanks go to John Bruin, Peter E. Siegler, M.D., and Arnold Melnick, D.O., for their infectious optimism and encouragement when I was just starting out as an editor.

I thank the many other kind souls who gave their time and effort while I was researching and writing this book, among them the following:

Frederick R. Mish, Ph.D., Editorial Director of Merriam-Webster Inc., for his erudition, patience, and unfailing good nature. William Wartman, for his invaluable counsel in the making of this book. For their generous assistance: Douglas Anderson, Hallie Baron, Jacques Barzun, Lee Bennett, Eli Chernin, Ph.D., Martin Cummings, M.D., Doris E. Davis, R.N., B.S.N., Rose DeWolf, Leonard S. Dreifus, M.D., Georgina Faludi, M.D., Joseph Farrell, Alan T. Forrester, Alice Hoersch, Ph.D., Charles R. Kalina, Lou Knecht, Robert B. Mehnert, Bernard L. Segal, M.D., Charles Swartz, M.D., Elizabeth J. Taylor, Elizabeth Van Lenten, Ph.D., and Barbara Williams.

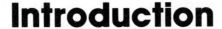

CHAPTER 1

Introduction

If one important message in this book could be condensed into a slogan, it would be that in usage anything does *not* go. The hazards of miscommunication are too great. In everyday conversation, little is lost if the conversers make mistakes in small talk. In medicine, mistakes can be injurious or even lethal. In the United Nations, the tone or translation of the resolution becomes world-important.

Highlighting other people's mistakes is an unorthodox way to write a book. Nevertheless, that's exactly what I've done. My own errors will, I hope, be tactfully pointed out or—better still for my editorial enrichment—gently corrected.

Many of the issues discussed are the result of queries addressed to me over the years as the author of the "Dear Edie" column on usage, a regular feature in the *American Medical Writers Association Journal* (*AMWA J*). I discovered that as the membership grew, different readers were asking the same questions I had discussed in previous columns, maybe years before. I also discovered in most instances that I had learned a great deal more in the interim about those selfsame subjects, so that my replies to the subsequent queries were more thoughtful and considered.

Almost all of the examples in this book, whether accurate, inaccurate, or unintentionally or inadvertently humorous, are taken from life—published material from medical, nursing, and pharmaceutical journals and books; health care and medical sections in newspapers and magazines; advertisements, brochures, and other advertising or public relations publications; and radio and television broadcasts. I have culled knotty problems, some not dealt with or difficult to locate in grammar, usage, or style books, but problems that confront writers and editors in their work every day—and I offer solutions. Editing, in particular, deals with subtleties and nuances.

The simple principles and explanations will probably be instantly intelligible to readers, whether they have had a good formal education or not. Self-education is all-important here, as in every other worthwhile endeavor.

The philosophy of English usage has always been important to me. Some examples and brief essays in this book deal with my feelings and beliefs on this subject.

Many topics overlap and therefore are discussed in more than one chapter. For this reason, we have attempted to keep the index as comprehensive as possible. Readers will be able to find what they're looking for quickly. As I've said so many times—and you can quote me—a book is only as good as its index. No one should have to scan an entire book to find one small allusion or reference.

If only part of a book entry is given, look in the Bibliography for the complete citation.

Three dictionaries, my mainstays, are referred to throughout this book—with affection and for convenience—by shorter designations: *Webster's Third New International Dictionary, Unabridged* as *Webster III* (*Webster Third*); *Dorland's Illustrated Medical Dictionary* as *Dorland's*; and *Stedman's Medical Dictionary* as *Stedman's*.

I have relied heavily on usage authorities and others whom I consider both reasonable and scholarly, as attested by the many quotations. To paraphrase Lucan and Sir Isaac Newton, we are all standing on the shoulders of giants.

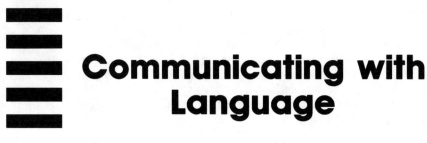

CHAPTER 2

Communicating with Language

True ease in writing comes from art, not chance,
As those move easiest who have learn'd to dance.
'Tis not enough no harshness gives offence,
The sound must seem an echo to the sense.

—Alexander Pope

Human beings were created curious. They had to venture from their caves to see what was over the next hill and the next. Once they found other tribes, they also found that gregariousness was better than hermitry. As soon as they made that discovery (give or take a few million years), the die was cast. To remain together they had to learn to communicate. Somewhere I read the following (paraphrased) list of five things that differentiate humans from the other animals. (If you know the source, please tell me.)

1. The opposing thumb
2. The discovery of fire
3. Brain development
4. Comprehension of the abstract; memory; and projection into the future
5. Language—written and spoken

Humans are the only beings that have the ability to communicate with language. The other animals make themselves understood, but without our kind of language.

Communication was born out of the need of humans to live together in reasonable harmony and to carry on commerce and other everyday transactions. No one knows how language arose, nor will we ever know.

As cities grew, and as trade and refinements in government progressed, it became more and more important for people of one nation to communicate intelligently with those of all other known countries.

TOWER OF BABEL CURSE

> And the whole earth was of one language, and of one speech. . . . And
> they said, 'Come, let us build a city, and a tower, with its top in heav-
> en . . .' And the Lord said: 'Behold, they are one people, and they
> have all one language; . . . and now nothing will be withholden from
> them . . . Come, let us go down, and there confound their language,
> that they may not understand one another's speech. . . .' Therefore
> was the name of it called Babel; because the Lord did there confound
> the language of all the earth . . .

The legend of the Tower of Babel (Genesis) seemed to have a moral: Humans must fail when they are so presumptuous as to try to touch
heaven. The punishment was to extend unto all generations, but it now
appears to have run its course.

Communication among all humans, imperfect though it may be, is
now possible. How? Radio, television, the telephone, and the computer.
These inventions have enabled humans to overcome the curse of the
Tower. We have bridged the oceans. We have reached the planets.

ENGLISH AS WORLD LANGUAGE

English is rapidly becoming the world language. In 1983 the
columnist Richard Reeves wrote: ". . . it seems likely that by the year
2000 there will be more nonnative English speakers than native. . . . In
this smaller world, you have to know English to 'keep up' with modern
developments—something like 80 percent of the world's technical
papers are first published in English. If you want to know—now!—what
is happening in computers or aviation, in accounting or rock music, you
have to know English."

The challenges inherent in this probability are breathtaking. Although the English language is idiomatic in the extreme, most of us
manage to make ourselves understood most of the time. It's the rest of
the time that I'm concerned about.

ILLITERACY OF THE EDUCATED AND MISEDUCATED

In conversation, almost anything goes. No one wants to kill
spontaneity. Even educated and informed people are not expected to
use perfect grammar in conversation. One simply cannot demand the
same standards in speaking as in writing. But serious writing—that's
another story.

The most important component of good communication is clarity.
As John Pittenger (formerly Secretary of Education of Pennsylvania)
and his staff put it, clarity begins at home.

In his advice on how to write clearly, Edward T. Thompson, Editor-in-Chief of the *Reader's Digest*, wrote: "Forget that old—and wrong—advice about writing to a 12-year-old mentality. That's insulting. But do remember that your prime purpose is to *explain* something, not prove that you're smarter than your readers." Better advice was never given.

To explain lucidly, one must learn how. There is a world of difference between "a little knowledge" and "a little learning." In *An Essay on Criticism*, Alexander Pope wrote:

A little learning is a dangerous thing;
Drink deep, or taste not the Pierian spring:
There shallow draughts intoxicate the brain,
And drinking largely sobers us again.

His exhortation was a plea for more and better education. He believed passionately in the beauty and value of learning. It matters little whether one is self-educated or has a formal education and a certificate to prove it. Some of us were fortunate enough to have had at least a good elementary and high school education; we were prepared to live and work in an ever more technologic and complex world.

Will there be well-educated, well-prepared American workers in the next century? This gravid problem now seems insoluble when one considers the poorly educated, poorly prepared students coming out of the schools in this generation.

The unfavorable prognosis may correlate with the purported "death of good English." In every age and every country, writers and other doomsayers have bemoaned the state of their particular language and have predicted its utter deterioration within the foreseeable future.

It is true that the lack of concern about excellence and standards in written expression in almost every segment of commerce has contributed heavily to the degradation of English. There are institutions and spheres of endeavor in which excellence and exactitude are ridiculed, frowned on, or irrationally feared: the schools, where "egghead" students are ostracized by their fellows; public relations and advertising, where correctness in usage is considered pretentious or undesirable ("the client likes it that way"—inaccurate); and television and radio, where "temperature" becomes "tempacher," "arrested" becomes "busted," "introduced" becomes "interduced," and the "big news" is a "copywritten" story about the latest insurrection.

Some journalists are—or were—under the impression that Rock Hudson underwent "six bypass surgeries" and that Marion Davies was the wife of William Randolph Hearst.

The columnist Sydney J. Harris wrote that it is "not the illiteracy of the uneducated that annoys me—you can't blame anyone for not knowing what has never been taught—but the illiteracy of the presumably educated in our society, and I include most college students and many teachers in this category. . . . People remember the dumbest, most trivial injunctions they learned in school, while neglecting the basic formation of language."

Jacques Barzun wrote that the "manhandling of words . . . helps to explain why the predominant fault of the bad English encountered today is not the crude vulgarism of the untaught but the blithe irresponsibility of the taught" (*On Writing, Editing, and Publishing*).

John Irving informs us that 90 percent of all writing consists of a thousand basic words. Other sources state that in everyday social transactions, most people use a vocabulary of perhaps 5,000 or 6,000 words. Few users or speakers of English are acquainted with more than one of ten words in the language, that is, 100,000 of a possible one million words.

Manuals and instructions for users of everything from shelving to computers are notorious for sounding as if they've been translated from other languages—and poorly, at that.

A Census Bureau report in 1986, based on a 1982 survey, concluded that 17 million to 21 million adults (over 20 years of age) in the United States were illiterate. The survey was commissioned by the U.S. Department of Education. The irony of this 13 percent illiteracy rate is that the agencies of government themselves are often guilty of using turgid, unintelligible language.

Bureaucratese, technologese, and other "-eses" (jargons) are responsible for the following barbarisms:

passive solar collector for *window*
valves of natural phenomenon for both *doors* and *windows*
energy management systems for *draperies* and *awnings*
instinctual for *instinctive*
precipitation situation for *rain* or *snow*
end-point for *result*
multiple for *many*
dialogue as a verb
interface for *talk*
input as a verb
intelligencewise, therapywise, and other dumb *-wise*s
time frame or period of time for *time*
great majority for *most*
impact as a verb
ongoing for *continuing*
suspicious for *questionable, equivocal,* or *inconclusive*
deaccessioned for *sold* or *disposed of*
oids for *corticosteroids*
in terms of for *in* or *with respect to*

basically
resulted from for *caused by*
minor breakthrough
counterproductive
demonstrated for *showed*
enhances for *increases*
minimizes for *decreases*
optimal for *best*
relatively when there is no antecedent or referent
pre-formatted
media as a catchall
chaise lounge for *chaise longue*
martyr by accident
correctional custodial facility for *guardhouse* or *jail*
automotive module attendants for *school bus drivers*

All of writing and editing consists of good judgment, subtleties, nuances, and shades of meaning. The *Stylebook/Editorial Manual of the AMA* (American Medical Association), 6th ed. (Littleton, Mass., Publishing Sciences Group, 1976), stated it elegantly:

> Exactitude, judgment, and knowledge are qualities of the professional copy editor. Since copy editing is both art and science, those who would take on its responsibilities must become disciplined in those qualities, the better to recognize when something is wrong or unclear, to judge whether the copy should be altered, and to know how to effect the correction or clarification.

Odds are that the student who has not read voraciously all of his or her life will not become a good writer. Writers learn to write first of all by reading.

Communication is not unilateral. There must be both a giving and a taking. Listening is the taking part. Mortimer Adler wrote that most people don't listen to what others are saying, either orally or in print. In conversation, most people just wait for a pause in the flow of language so that they can change the subject.

Listening to what is printed is even more difficult, because it's a solitary occupation requiring concentration and attentiveness. You should read someone else's article with all your attention. Read it for the rhythm of the sentences and the flow of thought. Don't read it with the idea of debating the author. Listen disinterestedly to all the author has to say. Start marshaling your own thoughts and mental rebuttal. Then write them down, if that was your original purpose in reading the article.

Many columnists and other writers complain that they receive letters from people who disagree not with what the authors have written but with what they have *not* written. More often than not, these readers misquote or read into the articles something that the author never intended—or wrote. Most painful of all to the writer is to have his or her motives completely misunderstood and to have readers ascribe malice or other sin when none exists.

PRESERVING THE LANGUAGE

If something is worth writing about and taking up room in medical journals, it clamors to be written and then published in lasting form. With permanent, acid-free paper and a little bit of luck, our printed works will outlast us. That thought may be unsettling, but it's exhilarating as well.

To halt the destruction of valuable writings, the United States National Library of Medicine (NLM), the largest health science library in the world, convened a task force in 1988. Its charge was to plan a campaign to "encourage and guide the use of acid-free paper in the publication of biomedical literature and to explore ways to implement the plan." Along with other library experts, Donald A. B. Lindberg, M.D., Director of the National Library of Medicine, believes that the best course to follow is to urge medical publishers to use permanent, acid-free paper for their publications in the first place.

Books printed on acid-free paper will last centuries, and those on other kinds of paper only a lifetime. Studies show that materials printed on acid-free paper and stored in clean air at freezing temperature could last several millennia.

Resolutions have been introduced in the Congress to implement the use of permanent, acid-free paper for all "permanently valuable Federal records" and to make this United States policy known to foreign governments and appropriate international agencies, since the acid paper problem is worldwide and materials imported by our libraries are printed on acid papers. There is little doubt that this legislation will be enacted.

Dr. Lois DeBakey, cochair (with Gerard Piel) of the Permanent Paper Task Force, voiced a caution: "With a clear danger of losing more than a century of the human record, can we afford to continue storing problems for the future?"

Gerald Piel informed his colleagues that the May 1948 issue of *Scientific American*, the first published under his management, is already showing signs of deterioration. He now realized, he said, that "my life's work is written in sand."

Good writers and speakers have no intention of allowing the deterioration of English despite the obstacles. The doomsaying was not necessary in Seneca's time, nor is it necessary now.

Jean Baptiste Lully, court composer in the reign of Louis XIV, had the chutzpah—on his death bed—to correct the attending priest's Latin.

Jacques Barzun, who epitomizes the good writer and editor, wrote that the "ideal writer would recast his own death sentence as he was reading it—if it was a bad sentence."

English is not dead—not while automobile manufacturers have enough respect for words and their meanings to name their models "Integra," "XL," and "Acura." The fact that the namers of the Acura used the root for "needle" rather than the one for "accurate" should not make us hypercritical. It's the thought that counts.

As long as there are humans, words will be better persuaders than anything else.

Good English is not dead, nor is it moribund—not while we lovers of the language, including the Jeremiahs and the Cassandras, continue our passionate efforts to conserve it. English is a living, working, wonderful language. It has power, vitality, richness, and beauty. Its artistry deserves preservation.

CHAPTER 3

Honest Mistakes and Miscomprehension

If we acknowledge that nobody's perfect, it follows that all of us make honest mistakes and sometimes fail to comprehend accurately. Some of these errors in writing and speaking come about because of homophony or similarity of meaning, or both. And some are caused by inadequate knowledge of medical terminology.

HOMOPHONY

Many common mistakes are made because of homophones, words that are pronounced alike but spelled differently.

> The governor declared marshal law.

That may be how the governor's announcement sounded, but what he meant was *martial* law.

> The president of the college seemed to the manor born.

The *manner* to which the president was born denotes an aristocratic *manner*, not the home in which she was born.

> The transition was smooth when the new hospital administration took over the reigns of power.

Reins, not *reigns*, because the metaphor properly refers to controlling a horse. Don't be led astray by "power."

> She gave an extra Phillip to the infusion line.

Phillip had nothing to do with it. The nurse probably gave the line an extra *fillip*, meaning in this instance a slight extra movement.
Fillip can also mean a rousing or stimulating agent, a trivial addition or minor embellishment, or a gesture made by the sudden forcible straightening of a finger curled up against the thumb. Its origin

is probably onomatopoeic or imitative, that is, intended to represent a natural sound.

EGREGIOUS ERRORS IN COLD PRINT

Honest mistakes are made because of inattentiveness or lack of comprehension; many others are, almost certainly, typographic errors. However, some may be due to lightweight intellectuality.

Here are some varied examples:

> Because the instructor used the Bell curve, the student received a much lower grade than she had expected.

This curve is named not for Alexander Graham Bell or any no-Bell but for the shape of the curve.

> Production of the film was halted when he underwent heart surgery and five heart bypasses.

Six operations altogether? Or a quintuple-vessel bypass operation? We'll never know from this Rock Hudson obituary. I speculate that five occluded blood vessels were bypassed. But your guess is as good as mine.

> The patient's main difficulty was aortic value disease.

In this instance the main difficulty was poor handwriting. Of course the problem was aortic *valve* disease.

> Pneumonia was the casual factor in her death.

What the writer meant here was that pneumonia, the *causal* factor, was responsible for the patient's death.

In my writing and editing, I always change *causal* to *causative*. Even casual typesetters never make a typo with that word.

> The 20 excluded patients are displayed in Table 2.

As long as it's not in Macy's window.

Good editing could obviate such absurdities. A proper way to structure that sentence is as follows: The 20 patients who were excluded from the study are listed in Table 2.

> Inscription on Oscar awarded to Spencer Tracy: Dick Tracy.

Keep your eye on the ball.

> Lice can sometimes be found in public hair.

No doubt.

> Classified advertisement: Medical asst.—For busy Ob-Gyn office. Lobotomy and prior medical office exp. required.

I don't believe that lobotomy is or should be a qualification for a medical assistantship.

> At the time of her death, she was a reference librarian at the Wilson Pubic Library.
>
> Many clinic patients are late for their appointments because they must take pubic transportation.

Both bits of information should be *public* knowledge.

> Government programs seek to curb the spread of AIDS by, among other things, encouraging people to refrain from premartial sex.

They also encourage people to refrain from *premarital* sex.

> His speech raised the ugly spectacle of war.

This misuse of *spectacle* by a well-known news commentator indeed raises a *specter*.

Unfortunately, broadcasters are seldom writers or editors, and writers or editors seldom become broadcasters.

> He was the discoverer of "Lucy," probably the oldest woman known to man.
>
> A 12-man jury, half of them women, will rule on the facts.

FREUDIAN SLIPS AND MISQUOTATION

> Cultural therapists know that music soothes the savage beast.

Thomas Congreve is often misquoted and his eminently quotable work misattributed (usually to Shakespeare). In his tragedy *The Mourning Bride*, he wrote:

> Music has [not hath] charms to soothe a [not the]
>   savage breast [not beast],
> To soften rocks, or bend a knotted oak.

He also wrote, in the same work:

> Heaven has no rage like love to hatred turned,
> Nor hell a fury like a woman scorned.

A feature column in the *New York Times* bore the headline "Play it again, Sam." The reference was to the movie *Casablanca*, in which Rick (Humphrey Bogart) tells the pianist to play the song he and his sweetheart (Ingrid Bergman) once shared: "Play it, Sam." Apparently the rhythmic addition of the word "again" is irresistible, though incorrect.

Shakespeare and the Bible are among the most often misquoted sources. Alexander Pope (see Chapter 2) runs them a close race.

Many quoters think that Shakespeare wrote "to gild the lily" in *King John*. Here's the actual expanded quotation:

> To gild refined gold, to paint the lily,
> To throw a perfume on the violet,
> To smooth the ice, or add another hue
> Unto the rainbow, or with taper-light
> To seek the beauteous eye of heaven to garnish,
> Is wasteful and ridiculous excess.

Makes a lot more sense that way, doesn't it?

Money is not the root of all evil. The following is the correct quotation from the first epistle of Paul to Timothy (6:7,10):

> For we brought nothing into this world, and it is certain we can carry nothing out. . . .
> For the love of money is the root of all evil . . .

The Bible doesn't say that pride goes before a fall. The proverb actually says:

> Pride goeth before destruction, and an haughty spirit before a fall.

Mark Twain (Samuel Clemens) never made that famous remark about the weather. It was made by Charles Dudley Warner, the associate editor of the *Hartford Courant*, in an editorial on August 24, 1897:

> Everybody talks about the weather, but nobody does anything about it.

The quotation is often mistakenly attributed to Twain, probably because he was the more famous of the two. He and Warner had collaborated on a book, *The Gilded Age* (1873).

MISCOMPREHENSION

> The clinical psychologist was able to resolve these inner-family disputes.

The writer of that sentence probably meant *intrafamily* disputes, since the context tells us that the psychologist was treating a particular family.

> There was a general lifting of spirits among homosexuals in lieu of the decreases in the number of cases of AIDS among homosexuals.

The writer undoubtedly meant *in light of*; presumably the error was caused by miscomprehension or lack of inclination to look things up. *In lieu of* means "instead of."

> Majewski was the penultimate person expected to join the ranks of the "most likely to succeed."

Penultimate is from the Latin *paene* or *pene*, meaning "almost" and *ultimus*, meaning "last." It means "next to the last," whether a person, a syllable in a word, or anything else.

The element *pen-* with the meaning "almost" should not be confused with the element *pen-* as in *penitentiary*, which stems from the Latin *poena*, "penalty" or "punishment." *Subpoena* means literally being "under penalty."

> Schwann's sheath was named for its founder.

This sheath, an anatomic part, was named after Theodor Schwann (1810–1882), the German anatomist and physiologist, who first described it in print.

The *schwannoma*, a neoplasm originating from *Schwann* cells (of the myelin sheath) of neurons, also termed neurofibroma or neurilemoma, is named for him, as was *schwannosis*. Several other anatomic parts or conditions are also named for him.

MIXED METAPHORS

As the ultimate expression of muddled thinking, this mixed metaphor, which appeared in a daily publication, deserves the booby prize:

> Even if Gorbachev is reined in, or toppled, the seeds he has sown in the Soviet mind and the changes he has already wrought will leave an indelible mark.

At least all the words are spelled right.

> A lot of water has gone under the dam since they decided to feather their nest with spurious accident claims.

Hmm. "Spurious" was a good choice of words. Too bad one can't say the same for the rest of the garbled metaphor.

In one of his picaresque novels, Ian Fleming wrote:

> Bond's knees, the Achilles heel of all skiers, were beginning to ache.

Theodore Bernstein called these jumbled figures of speech "mixaphors."

Writers should guard against intermixing metaphors or images that don't belong together.

TYPOGRAPHIC ERRORS

> By contrast, many Englishmen pass less than 150 grams of hard stools a day and then may take between three and five days to traverse the alimentary canal.

One hopes that in this convoluted (to match the alimentary canal) sentence, *then* is a typographic error and should have read *they.* However, that change would hardly remedy the sentence's murkiness.

> The cardiologist had seen him regularly in recent years because of a trial fibrillation.

A dry run for the real thing? Of course this should have read "because of *atrial* fibrillation."

> People engaged in hard physical labor do not have a deceased risk of colorectal cancer.

There is no question that this was a typographic error; it appeared in a popular column on health written by a respected physician. The editor (if any) and the proofreader (if any) must have been absent that day.

> The factor most responsible for baldness is generic.

Medical knowledge tells us that some types of baldness are inherited, and are thus *genetic.*

> The x-rays for 9 patients revealed labor pneumonia.

Transposed vowels. "*Lobar* pneumonia" was what it should have read. Perhaps this was a Freudian slip made by a typist in an agency handling workmen's compensation.

SCRAMBLED MEDICAL KNOWLEDGE

> Two patients underwent an anaphylactic response.

They *had* anaphylactic responses. Patients may *undergo* tests or procedures.

> Classified advertisement in the Help Wanted section: The laboratory applicant should be familiar with mixing acids and preferably have a background in tight trading.

This grievous error (it was a real advertisement) was made because the order had been taken over the phone. The ad-taker heard "tight trading"; the ad-giver mistakenly assumed that everyone knows what *titrating* is.

> Medical students take the Hypocratic Oath on graduation.

Although the pronunciation is the same, the oath is correctly spelled *Hippocratic*, after Hippocrates (c. 460–c. 377 B.C.), the great physician and teacher at the medical school on the Greek island of Cos. He is known as the "father of medicine," primarily because of his principled approach to the practice of medicine. The oath, of which there are several versions, is generally attributed to Hippocrates; it prescribes a code of ethics for those about to enter the practice of medicine.

> Several patients wore halter monitors around the clock.

No wonder the writer made this error. The words *halter* and *Holter* sound almost exactly alike. Nonmedical writers might think that these monitors are worn around the neck as well as around the clock. But it is not so. Electrodes on the patient's body are attached to a *Holter monitor*, an electrocardiographic recorder, worn over the shoulder or on a belt at the waist. After 24 hours, the monitor and electrodes are removed and the recording tape is read by computer in the heart station.
This monitor was invented by the engineer Norman Holter.

> The disorder known as Lugerics disease gets even more publicity when a celebrity dies of it.

The strangely familiar-sounding disease referred to, which will not be found in any book of medical eponyms, is meant to be *Lou Gehrig's disease*, amyotrophic lateral sclerosis.

> Frank Peritonitis was a famous Greek physician and athlete.

The student, who had hoped to take premedical courses, flunked this multiple-choice test.

> Physicians administer barbiturates to near-drowning victims to control inner-cranial pressure and other problems.

As opposed to outer cranial pressure? What was meant here was *intracranial pressure*, pressure within the cranium. This error reminds me of the person who pronounces "introduce" as "innerduce" or "interduce."

> The Propriety Association is a trade group representing manufacturers of over-the-counter drugs.

What kind of naughty group would the Nonpropriety Association be?

PROOFREADING

In 1977 Max Lerner wrote in a newspaper article that "we admonish the young to say exactly what they think. But we know, as writers, that often we are surprised by what comes out. How will we know what we think until we see what we have written?"

And how will we know what we have written until we proofread what we have written?

Typographic errors are perhaps the easiest ones to spot and to correct. Other kinds of mistakes require editorial skill, greater concentration, and closer examination. Writers should make an invariable practice of proofreading the final version of a manuscript before submitting it to a journal or publisher. No one is perfect—not the writer and not the typist.

Often, when one error is corrected, another one is introduced. Every proofreader is aware of this possibility and is on the alert for proximal typos in published material.

In *A History of Judaism*, Daniel J. Silver wrote that the "*Talmud* had warned the scribes to be careful [in describing God's revelation]: 'Yours is sacred work; by leaving out or adding a single letter you can destroy the whole world.'"

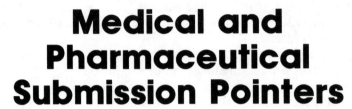

CHAPTER 4

Medical and Pharmaceutical Submission Pointers

ABSTRACTS

Abstracts of articles should not ordinarily appear in lists of references, unless the publication permits it. These are some of the reasons why *Index Medicus* does not publish citations of abstracts:

IM's policy is to cite journal articles of a substantive nature. Abstracts are not of a substantive nature.

It would be repetitious. Some of the articles are ultimately published in *IM* as full articles, which, unlike abstracts, are cited in *IM*.

The sheer volume of abstracts makes it almost impossible to cite them properly. Abstracts from proceedings on the topics of the societies are not cited individually, but the proceedings as a whole might be.

AGONIST, ANTAGONIST

In pharmacology, an *agonist* is a substance that acts with, enhances, or potentiates a specific activity. W. S. Haubrich wrote that "when referring to muscles, an agonist is a prime mover, and its antagonist is a muscle having the opposite effect. In physiological terms, an agonist is a stimulant to a specific action, while an antagonist blocks or counteracts the stimulus. Histamine, for example, is an agonist when it stimulates the secretion of hydrochloric acid by the parietal or oxyntic cells of the stomach; cimetidine, acting as an H_2-receptor antagonist, blocks this action."

Naloxone is another antagonist. It competes with morphine for receptor sites in the brain and other tissues, thereby keeping the morphine from binding to the receptors and having an adverse effect.

APGAR SCORE

The Apgar in *Apgar score* is not an acronym. The eponymous test is named for Virginia Apgar (1909–1974), the world-renowned American physician-anesthesiologist who devised it and thereby revolutionized neonatology.

Dr. L. Joseph Butterfield, of Children's Hospital, Denver, has come up with a mnemonic device for recalling the five Apgar criteria: *a*ppearance, *p*ulse, *g*rimace, *a*ctivity, and *r*espiration, thus making APGAR an acronym after all.

AZT, RETROVIR, AND AIDS

The Burroughs Wellcome Company of Research Triangle Park, North Carolina, is the manufacturer of Retrovir, its agent active against the human immunodeficiency virus (HIV).

Zidovudine (pronounced zy-doe-view-deen, accent on doe) was formerly known as azidothymidine (AZT). The Burroughs Wellcome immunosuppressant drug Imuran (generic name, azathioprine) is also called AZT in some countries. Therefore, Burroughs Wellcome assigned a new trade name to zidovudine—Retrovir.

Azidothymidine was initially synthesized in 1964 by Jerome Horwitz, of the Michigan Cancer Foundation, as a potential treatment for cancer, but studies were abandoned soon after because the compound showed no activity against animal cancer.

In the early 1980s, Burroughs Wellcome resynthesized azidothymidine and sent it to the laboratories at the National Cancer Institute, the Food and Drug Administration, and Duke University for independent testing to determine its effectiveness against the human immunodeficiency virus (HIV). They determined early in 1985 that azidothymidine was indeed active against HIV in vitro.

Burroughs Wellcome submitted an IND (Investigational New Drug) Application to the FDA on June 14, 1985 for permission to use the compound in patients with AIDS or advanced AIDS-related complex (ARC). In the meanwhile, the company tooled up for more rapid synthesis of the compound (the manufacture begins with the chemical thymidine, a naturally occurring but rare substance, and ordinarily takes about seven months). One week after submission of the IND application, the FDA granted permission for clinical testing of azidothymidine in humans. Thereupon, Burroughs Wellcome supplied the compound free of charge to almost 5,000 patients enrolled in the studies.

Clinical testing showed that among other advantages, this compound could cross the blood-brain barrier, an important finding because the HIV causes neurologic disease.

In March 1987, after a breathtakingly short (four months) review of a New Drug Application (NDA), the U.S. Food and Drug Administration approved the Retrovir brand of zidovudine.

The rest is medical, pharmaceutical, and public health history, and that history is still being made.

BACTERIA

Most foreign terms (primarily Latin and Greek) that are used in everyday medical writing containing the ligatures æ and œ have been simplified or anglicized to conform with the pronunciation. Transliteration into English from other languages is always difficult, especially from a non-Roman alphabet.

Amoeba and *haemorrhage* lend themselves readily to the simpler *ameba* and *hemorrhage*. Some medical associations and specialists (some orthopaedists and paediatricians, for instance) retain the ancient spelling.

Logic would seem to call for the anglicization of such difficult spellings as those of bacteria and other microorganisms. However, much as we might want to simplify, we must resist that impulse. *Haemophilus influenzae* is the proper name for that bacterium. Although *Hemophilus* is pronounced exactly the same way, the official spelling is still *Haemophilus*.

As a colleague, an expert in microbiology, explained, you wouldn't change the spelling of your own or a friend's name, would you? No more should you change the established, official names of microorganisms, as described in exquisite detail in *Bergey's Manual of Determinative Bacteriology*, the bible. These names are invariable, at least until they are officially changed or updated.

Note that full names of bacteria are italicized (underlined in typing) and that the first element is always capitalized; the secondary element is lowercase.

For a helpful condensed discussion of the written forms of organisms, consult the eighth edition of the *American Medical Association Manual of Style* ("Organisms," pp. 242–244).

CADUCEUS

Two kinds of wands—*caducei*—are often mistaken one for the other. They are not interchangeable. One kind of *caduceus*—the Latin adaptation of Greek terms signifying a herald's staff—is a stylized representation of a wand with two serpents curled around it and with wings atop the staff. This was Mercury's wand.

Statues and other representations of Mercury (Hermes in Greek mythology), the mischievous messenger of the gods and the Roman god of commerce, show him in flight with winged heels and cap and carrying a two-serpented caduceus. A national long-distance florist company uses such a statue as its logo (logotype) to emphasize the swiftness of its service.

The wooden staff of Aesculapius, the mythic Greco-Roman god of medicine, has a branched top and only one snake entwined around it. The Aesculapian staff is the official insigne of the World Medical Association, the American Medical Association, and some branches of the United States armed forces. Other branches of the armed forces use the double-serpented caduceus as their insigne. Why they do so is a mystery to me, although it has been suggested that the wings atop the caduceus symbolize the wings of the air forces.

Nonetheless, there is a mythologic connection between Mercury and Aesculapius. Apollo, the god of health, presented a wand to Mercury, to be used for healing. As for Aesculapius, when Apollo discovered that his lover, Coronis, who was carrying his child, had been unfaithful, he killed her and removed the child, Aesculapius, by caesarean section.

Greek and Roman mythology teems with stories about health deities.

Incidentally, the two daughters of Aesculapius were Hygeia and Panacea. All three mythical characters are invariably depicted in contemporary representations with compassionate, wise faces.

CAPITALIZATION IN HEADINGS

Many newspapers use *library style* (also called *sentence style*) in their headlines, and many medical journals use it in the titles of articles. Library style is capitalizing the first word in a head and, of course, any proper names, nouns, or adjectives; all other words start with lowercase letters.

The rules, when library style is *not* used, are simple:

In titles of poems, chapters, parts, books, and all other such material, the first *and last* words are always capitalized, no matter what part of speech the last word may be. All important words should also be capitalized, even if they are only two letters long (*Is, Be*). Nouns, pronouns, verbs, adjectives, and adverbs should always be capitalized. Other parts of speech, such as articles, prepositions, and coordinating conjunctions (*or, but, and*) are ordinarily not capitalized unless they are the last words in the titles. The word *to*, whether preposition or part of an infinitive, is not capitalized.

Prepositions containing more than four letters may or may not be capitalized; many authors make it a rule to use lowercase for all prepositions, no matter how many letters they may be, just to keep life simple.

Some publishers and others prefer to capitalize all prepositions with four or more letters: *Over, Through, Before, Between*. Either style is "right." Here house style or consistency is the watchword. Decide on a style at the outset and follow it faithfully throughout any one piece of work.

Standing By for Further Word from the Department of Pathology

In this example, *By* is initial-cap because it is actually a part of the verb, what is called a *fused verb form*, in which the less important word would ordinarily be an adverb.

Use initial-cap for the first word that comes after a colon or a dash in a title, subtitle, or subhead, no matter what part of speech it is.

Hyphens in titles are also discussed in this chapter.

Cesarean, Caesarean, cesarean, or caesarean?

There is no need to capitalize this obstetric term. Contrary to popular belief, it did not originate and could not have originated with the birth of Julius Caesar.

This surgical operation—cesarean or caesarean section—had been performed for many centuries before Gaius Julius Caesar was born, but only on a mother's dead body, never on a live woman. However, for Julia, Julius's mother, that was ancient history—she lived for many years after his birth.

Julius might have been named Caesar because of his blue-gray eyes (the Latin word for bluish gray is *caesicius*) or because, as the legend goes, he was born with a full head of hair (the Latin for long-haired is *caesariatus*).

The term *caesarian section* is most likely from *sectio caesaria*, a Medieval Latin phrase meaning exactly the same as in English, a surgical operation or cutting through of the walls of the abdomen and uterus to deliver the offspring of a human or an animal. *Caesum* is the past participle of *caedo* (I cut).

The German word for this operation is *Kaiserschnitt* ("imperial" or "emperor's" cut). Caesar, kaiser, and czar (tsar) all mean "king" or "emperor."

CF.

This abbreviation stands for *confer*, a Latin word meaning "compare." It usually precedes a word that has a meaning different from the defined word.

Colleague. Cf. cohort

The *cf.* is a signpost that the following word—in this instance *cohort*—has a meaning different from that of *colleague*. True verbophiles or verbomaniacs will immediately look up *cohort* to fix the differentiation between the two meanings in their minds.

COLUMN HEADS IN TABLES

When every item in a table or a column is a percentage, there is no need to repeat the percent symbol (%) after each item. The column head could include the percent symbol in parentheses after the absolute number of patients, thus killing two columns with one stone. The column head would then read: "No. of Subjects (%)," meaning the number of subjects and the percentage of subjects in that particular category. Table 1 is preferable to Table 2.

(Fictitious examples)

Table 1. Adverse events necessitating discontinuation of the study

Event	No. of subjects (% of group)	
	Placebo	Drug
Anemia (hemoglobin < 8 g/dL) necessitating transfusion	1 (0.2)	5 (1.1)
Neutropenia*	7 (1.6)	8 (1.8)
Nausea	1 (0.2)	15 (3.3)
*Absolute neutrophil count < 750 cells/mm^3.		

Table 2. Adverse events necessitating discontinuation of the study

Event	No. of subjects	
	Placebo	Drug
Anemia (hemoglobin < 8 g/dL) necessitating transfusion	1 (0.2%)	5 (1.1%)
Neutropenia*	7 (1.6%)	8 (1.8%)
Nausea	1 (0.2%)	15 (3.3%)
*Absolute neutrophil count < 750 cells/mm^3.		

CONSISTENCY OF TERMS

Numerals, whether roman or arabic, should be consistent for the same term, at least within the same piece of work.

> Type 1 agents are local anesthetics; type IA agents prolong conduction and refractoriness.

That sentence should contain either 1 and 1A or I and IA. In most instances, it should be "type 1A," since the roman numeral is sometimes read as a capital *I*. For this reason, I usually spell out *intravenous* in preference to abbreviating it IV or i.v.; *intravenous* can never be misread. "IV" could be misread as roman numeral four.

After first mention, *intravenous* may be abbreviated, since "I.V." (complete with periods) is a well-understood and accepted term in English.

Blood coagulation factors are expressed in roman numerals, with the activated form indicated by an *a* after the numeral. Some writers in neoplastic diseases prefer to use fuller forms: antihemophilic globulin or thromboplastinogen rather than factor VIII and fibrin stabilizing factor, or fibrinase, rather than factor XIII. Platelet factors are expressed in arabic numerals. The principal factor, platelet factor 3, is the generic term for certain phospholipids.

Another possible glitch is use of the capital *L* in the chemical abbreviation or symbol for hydrochloride: "Tocainide HCL is an antiarrhythmic agent." Of course that should be HCl, with a lowercase letter *l* (sometimes misinterpreted as the numeral 1 by typists, word processor operators, and readers).

CROSS AND HYPHENS

According to *Webster III, cross section* (as a noun) is not hyphenated, but *cross-section* (as a verb) is. *Cross-sectional* (adjective) is hyphenated, as are *cross-pollinate, cross-purpose, cross-question, cross-reaction, cross-reference* (noun and verb), *cross-resistance*, and *cross-tolerance*.

Crossroad is written solid, as is *crossword. Crossover* as a noun is solid, but as a verb it is two words: *cross over. Cross product* is also two words.

DANA-FARBER CANCER INSTITUTE

The correct name of this institute is Dana-Farber (not Dana Farber) Cancer Institute. The work of Sidney Farber, M.D. and his colleagues with chemotherapy had achieved the first complete remissions in children with some forms of leukemia.

In 1947 Farber, with the collaboration of the Variety Club of New England and the help of the Boston Braves (and, after the Braves moved to Milwaukee, the Boston Red Sox), founded the institute as the Children's Cancer Research Foundation.

To honor its founder, the institute was renamed the Sidney Farber Cancer Institute in 1976; the name was changed again, in 1983, to Dana-Farber Cancer Institute, to recognize the long-standing support of Charles A. Dana, a New York industrialist, and his Dana Foundation.

The institute, a teaching affiliate of Harvard Medical School, is one of 20 federally designated comprehensive cancer centers in the United States.

DESCRIBING TECHNIQUES AND METHODS

Readers are gratified when the writer does not burden or weary them with unnecessary details about certain techniques and methods used in the investigation. If a description of the particular methods used to gather the writer's data has been previously published, state simply that the "Pate technique is described elsewhere." The writer could reinforce the information by documenting the technique in the text with a reference number and then including the previously published descriptive article in the list of references.

DECIMALS AND LESS THAN ONE

When units are written out, use the singular for quantities of 1 or less: 0.25 gram (*not* grams); 0.2 second (two-tenths of *a* second).

DECIMALS AND TABLES

In tables, the decimal points (whether or not percentages) should be aligned, and all the items in a column should have the same number of numerals (places) after the decimal; for a whole number, write one or two zeros after the decimal. Whole numbers in a column are aligned on the right:

82.1	1,258
6.3	324
11.8	25
52.9	6
26.0	2,079

DECIMALS THAT CAN KILL

In the old days (B.C.—before computers), prescriptions filled at hospital pharmacies were recorded on certain duplicative forms. Some physicians are or were in the habit of writing a decimal point and a zero after whole numbers, for example, 2.0 for 2. If the decimal point didn't register on the copy of the order, the prescription would read 20 mg instead of 2.

You can imagine the mischief this could cause with the dose of digoxin or other therapeutic but potentially lethal agents. Today, the accuracy of numbers in a manuscript depends on the alertness, intelligence, skill, and experience of the word processor operator, as well as the prescriber's handwriting.

Ordinarily there is no difference in medical practice between 2.0 mg and 2 mg. However, the science or medical writer should be aware that the zeros after a decimal point in some instances may be "significant digits"—denoting the preciseness of the measurement—and therefore may warrant inclusion.

D.M.D.

This abbreviation, which is New Latin, stands for Dentariae Medicinae Doctor, Doctor of Dental Medicine.

DOUBLE-SPACING OF MANUSCRIPTS

The importance of leaving plenty of white space in manuscripts cannot be overestimated. Typists should be instructed to DOUBLE-SPACE OR TRIPLE-SPACE EVERYTHING IN A MANUSCRIPT: quotations or excerpts, column heads in tables, and *especially* the list of references, legends for figures, and tables. These last three segments are usually the most heavily edited portions, so generous margins and white space are needed for editorial and production notations.

Remember that if a word is in boldface or italics *and* capitals, the editor needs space for *four* lines under the word—a squiggly horizontal line for boldface, or a straight horizontal line for italics, two additional straight horizontal lines for small capitals, and three additional straight horizontal lines to indicate large capitals.

Some typists believe that because something will ultimately appear in fine print anyway, it should be single-spaced in the manuscript. Nothing is more likely to make an editor groan. Leave the specifications of small print and other details of production and design to the people at the publisher's house. The publisher will invariably and inevitably change your style to the house style in all respects.

You can't ever go wrong by double-spacing or triple-spacing a manuscript, and the editor will remember you in her or his will.

ENDEMIC, EPIDEMIC, PANDEMIC, EPIZOOTIC

These terms are often confused. Or at least, the people who have to use them are confused.

Endemic refers to a disease or condition present in a population or region all the time.

Epidemic refers to a disease, condition, or outbreak that occurs suddenly and in great numbers, far beyond the expectable numbers. Sometimes it is used to refer to a disease brought in from another region.

Pandemic refers to a disease or condition that affects an extensive area or is extensively epidemic over a large region, hemisphere, or continent (or the world).

Epizootic refers to a disease or condition affecting many animals simultaneously, and is the animal counterpart of epidemic. (Greek *epi-*, upon; *demos*, the people; *zoon*, animal.)

EPONYMS

Eponym is from the Greek *epi*, meaning "on" or "upon," and *onyma*, meaning "name." An eponym is "one for whom or which something is named or supposedly named." In medical contexts, eponyms are most often used in the common names (nicknames) of diseases, disorders, syndromes, tests, anatomic parts, reagents, or methods.

Some authorities and journals discourage this use of eponyms, preferring to use more precise, descriptive (and usually much more cumbersome) medical terms. There may be, they say, more than one kind of disease or syndrome with that particular person's name. Their logic is unassailable.

The busy writer could have it both ways: Just as acronyms should be spelled out initially and thereafter abbreviated, the writer could use the eponymous common name at the outset, with the more descriptive medical name given in parentheses, and then use the nickname throughout the work.

In most instances, euphony governs the use or nonuse of the apostrophe and *s* in eponyms. Either Down or Down's syndrome is correct; so are Graves' or Graves's disease and Ringer or Ringer's solution.

The eponymous term for one highly malignant tumor (*nephroblastoma* is one formal synonym) is taken from the renowned German surgeon Max Wilms (1867–1918), who described it in an 1899 publication.

The following examples are incorrect:

> The introduction of a normal human chromosome 11 into murine Wilm's tumor cells completely suppressed their ability to form tumors.

> The results of urine cytology testing in children with Wilm's tumor are generally normal.

Wilms, Wilms', and Wilms's are all correct. Wilm's is not, since the physician's name was Wilms.

One "rule" is that when the anatomic part, syndrome, disease, or other eponymous term contains the name of more than one person, the apostrophe and *s* are not used: Wolff-Parkinson-White syndrome;

Zollinger-Ellison syndrome; Neubauer-Fischer test; Miller-Abbott (or Abbott-Miller) tube; Starr-Edwards valve.

In one-name or one-person eponyms, sometimes the possessive apostrophe and *s* are used and sometimes they are not. Here tradition and your favorite medical dictionaries are the arbiters. Of course, one should make sure that it is indeed a one-person eponym: Argyll Robertson sign (pupil or syndrome, or reflex iridoplegia) is named for Douglas Moray Cooper Lamb Argyll Robertson (1837–1909); however, most dictionaries of eponyms point the reader to "Robertson's syndrome" if "Argyll Robertson syndrome" is sought. Similarly, Ferguson Smith's epithelioma honors J. Ferguson Smith. Hyphens are sometimes erroneously inserted in these names.

Eponymous terms are heavily weighted in favor of the physician who originally described the particular disease rather than the patient who had it. One famous exception is *HeLa cell*, an eponym for a strain of robust, rapidly proliferating cancer cells cultured in 1951 by George Gey, of Johns Hopkins University, from a patient known variously as *He*len *La*ne, *He*len *La*rson, and *He*nrietta *La*cks. The offspring of her cells lived on, although she died that same year, to be used as the standard cell in oncology laboratories all over the world for testing new culture media or techniques.

HeLa is not only an eponym but also an acronym.

ERRORS IN LISTS OF REFERENCES

Studies show that half to three quarters of all references in lists of references contain at least one erroneous item. A misfingering on the keyboard, an error in one digit of a year, or a misspelled name will make it a difficult and time-consuming task to find the original printed article.

HYPHENS IN TITLES

Hyphens sometimes present a problem in headings and titles when initial-cap style (and not library style) is used.

The first part of a hyphenated term in a heading should always be capitalized: All-American Surgical Team Off to Europe. Both elements of a nonce or temporary compound term that would not otherwise be hyphenated should be capitalized: Endothelium-Mediated; Full-Term Babies; High-Fiber Diets, Diagnosis-Related Group.

If the compound term is always hyphenated, the element following the hyphen should be lowercase: Cardiology in the Twenty-first Century; Problems in Self-esteem and Body Image; Decision-making as a Course of Study; Double-spacing Manuscripts.

In longer hyphenated terms or phrases, the rule concerning capitalization of only important words stands: Catch-as-Catch-Can Administration; Cat-and-Mouse Game in the House—and the Senate.

ISBN

This initialism, which is found on the copyright page of almost every book one sees today, stands for *International Standard Book Number*. It contains digits assigned by the publisher in accordance with an arbitrary international numbering system. For example, in (fictitious) ISBN 0-111-22222-3, the first number, 0, represents the group (that is, language or country); the second set of numbers, 111, indicates the publisher; the third set, 22222, identifies the individual book. The last number is the "check digit," for computer purposes, that is, to automatically disclose errors in the preceding group.

JUSTIFIED LINES IN MANUSCRIPTS

Many medical journal and book publishers ask writers to use unjustified (ragged or uneven) right margins in their manuscripts. This request may puzzle many book readers, and some authors as well, who are accustomed to seeing rigidly even right margins in their manuscripts and who are consequently displeased with seemingly unesthetic ragged right margins.

This initial feeling of displeasure is soon dispelled when they understand the main reason for uneven right margins: The publisher's production people cannot make an accurate count of words in a manuscript, whether article or book, on justified lines (lines with words spaced in procrustean mode, to align with a rigid right margin).

The prospective author should be aware of the capabilities and limitations of word processors, software, and word processor operators. Some operators use only the block form of paragraphing (no indention)—setting tabs (tabular stops) is too time-consuming for them. This practice causes editors to shake their heads in despair; they can't tell whether the top line on a new page really starts a paragraph or just a new sentence.

LEONARDO DA VINCI

In alphabetizing or indexing, the name of this Renaissance man is usually listed with the *V*'s. Sometimes, however, his name is listed under *L*. The reason is that *da Vinci* refers to his hometown, Vinci, in Tuscany. *Da* is Italian for "from," "by," or "at."

Aside from being one of the greatest medical illustrators of all time, Leonardo was an architect, an engineer, a painter, a scientist, a sculptor, and a writer. His magnificent anatomic drawings, more than 1,500 of them, are still used (despite the errors) and are reproduced over and over, sometimes as a logotype for medicine or anatomy. The medical historian Felix Marti-Ibañez called him the "most creative genius of all time."

LITER

At one time *liter* was not abbreviated (10 g/liter) except in compound terms, when it was lowercase: milliliter, ml; deciliter, dl. That was because in typing, lowercase *l* often looks exactly the same as the number 1. In fact, on some typewriters and other machines they are interchangeable.

In most American medical journals and books, the convention is now to use uppercase *L* for "liter" or "liters," whether after a virgule (meaning "per") or in prefixed terms: 10 g/L; mL; dL. Follow the house style. When it is not preceded by numerals in text, *liter* should be spelled out.

The word *liter* is from the French *litre*, out of the medieval Latin and Greek *litra*, a weight or coin.

For numerophiles: a liter is approximately equal to 1.057 quarts (liquid); 0.908 quart (dry); and 61.02 cubic inches.

LOGOTYPE

Logo is a short term for *logotype*, a single piece of type. It usually includes the name of a company or an advertiser's trademark and some distinctive graphic art.

Often the logotype bears a trademark ™, service mark ˢᴹ, or copyright registry circle ©.

MORBIDITY, MORTALITY RATES

The *American Medical Association Manual of Style* points out that *morbidity* refers to the condition of being diseased. The "*morbidity rate* (or *attack rate*) is the number of cases of a specific disease divided by the total population at risk for that disease."

Mortality refers to the number of deaths from a certain disorder or disease. The *mortality rate* is the "number of deaths in a particular population divided by the size of that population at the same time."

> The mortality from stroke is vastly underrated by the lay public.
> Cardiovascular disease accounts for a high mortality rate in the United States.

NUMBERS AND CONSISTENCY

In a medical or other scientific context, journalism rules are inappropriate, including the one relating to numbers. In newspapers and similar publications, numbers through nine (sometimes ten) are spelled out, with arabic numbers being used for 10 and numbers larger than 10.

One problem with the journalistic practice is ambiguity:

> Epidemiologists estimated that as many as three to 9,000 in the community had been exposed to the fungus.

Does that mean three or 3,000? The writer must be queried.

In expressions containing a percentage, the % symbol or the word *percent* or *per cent* should always follow *each* number in such expressions, even when the numbers are separated by a dash, as in a range. The number in a percentage should always be written as a number, never spelled out.

> The protein-binding values of dipyridamole have been reported to range from 91 percent to 99 percent.

Some readers may argue that there is no possibility of ambiguity in that sentence. But that argument fails to take into account that some day there will be such a possibility in another term if the symbol is omitted from the first element. Therefore, the best practice is to *always* insert the symbol in *each* element.

Even when the house style of a journal is to spell out numerals through nine, numbers—not words—should be used for *all* numbers from 1 to infinity in a paragraph that is peppered with numbers. This practice simplifies life for both writer and reader. I'm glad I adopted it at the outset of my editing career.

OXYGEN

Don't expect everyone to know the chemical symbol for oxygen, O_2. With that realistic lack of expectation, make sure that when the word processor text is printed out, the O is a capital letter O and not the number zero, 0.

PERSONAL COMMUNICATIONS

Personal communications, whether letters or telephonic or other oral communications, should not be included in lists of references, since they are not documented or public, and so cannot be easily authenticated. They can be described in the text either as a full sentence or as a fragment in parentheses, immediately after the piece of attributed information:

> In a letter received from Jean LeBeau, D.O. in January 1987, he stated . . .
>
> In a conversation in March 1988, Hermano Arias Aguilar, M.D. reported that . . .
>
> Our findings in this aspect of the study agree with those of Galena Radetzky, Ph.D. (written communication, September 1989).

Note that academic degrees are included in the attribution. Dates of communications are essential.

pH VALUE

In 1909 the Danish chemist Søren Peter Lauritz Sørensen, Ph.D. invented a handy way to measure and record acidity or alkalinity of solutions (the Sørensen scale). He called it the pH value, which is expressed in numbers from 0 to 14 and denotes the negative logarithm of the concentration of the hydrogen ion: The larger the number, the lower the concentration of hydrogen ion.

It's much easier to say "pH 7" (neutrality) than to use the expression "hydrogen ion concentration of 10^{-7} (10 to the minus seventh power) moles per liter."

PIXEL

Pixel, a term used in television, computer work, and imaging (NMRI, nuclear magnetic resonance imaging, or just MRI), is short for *picture element*, the tiny points on a screen. The sharpness and detail of the monitor image depend on the number of pixels. An image or picture with 250,000 pixels would be sharp and clear; one with only 50,000 would be grainy and diffuse.

Pixel, sometimes shortened to *pix*, should not be confused with *pix*, a *Variety* abbreviation for picture (movie), or with a *pyx*, which in an ecclesiastical context is a container to hold the sacrament, and in a secular context a chest used in a British or American mint to hold sample coins for subsequent testing and assay.

POINTS AND PERIODS

Periods are ordinarily used in pharmacy terms such as b.i.d., t.i.d., and p.o. to avoid even the faintest possibility of misunderstanding a prescription or a patient's chart. As discussed under "Decimals That Can Kill," occasionally one reads a sensational news story about the lethal results of misreading a decimal point in a dose or the percentages in an infusion.

In pharmaceutical practice, "O.U." could mean either *oculus uterque* (each eye) or *oculi unitas* (both eyes, together). If the practitioner's handwriting is not clear, the written "ou" or "O.U." could be read as "a.u." or "A.U.," which means "each ear" or "both ears."

Another abbreviation that is often misinterpreted from handwriting is "q.d.," (every day), especially when the period after "q." is read as an "i," making this abbreviation read "q.i.d." (four times a day).

"O.D.," *oculus dexter* (right eye), is sometimes misread as "once a day." Such instructions should always be spelled out. A handwritten "U" (for units) especially lends itself to misinterpretation as a zero, a mistake that could lead to death by inadvertence.

There is a difference between 2 and 2.0 when one needs to use significant digits to denote the degree of preciseness in measurement; however, in prescribing, there is no difference between 2.0 mg and 2 mg.

All in all, the trend in medical practice should be toward writing prescription instructions in English words rather than Latin abbreviations. Then the pharmacist would have to worry only about the handwriting.

Carelessness may cause misunderstanding when a writer is hurried or harried. A case in point is sloppiness in placing the decimal in the wrong place:

> The rate of stenotic worsening, 11.5% per month for restenosis versus 13% per month for disease progression, was significantly different.

An alert editor noted that the difference between these two figures is *not* significant. The second percentage should have been 1.3%, which *is* a statistically significant difference.

See also the section on periods in Chapter 7, "Punctuation."

PROPRIETARY AND NONPROPRIETARY NAMES

Because it usually takes about 10 years and $130 million or more to research, develop, and market a new product, pharmaceutical manufacturers are justifiably proprietary about these preparations. *Proprietary* is no pun. That's the noun and the adjectival term used to designate drugs, agents, chemicals, medications, substances, and other preparations that manufacturers have an exclusive right—for a legally prescribed and defined time—to call their own.

To differentiate a *proprietary* name (also called a trademark or brand name) from a *nonproprietary* name (OTC, or "over-the-counter" preparations), the proprietary names are always written with an initial capital letter: Inderal, Librium. Nonproprietary or generic names are written with an initial lowercase letter: thalidomide; chlordiazepoxide hydrochloride; propranolol hydrochloride.

Public relations and advertising agencies have their own special rules about using a trademark or registry circle with a proprietary name. People who work in these fields should be conversant with their particular agencies' standards; there are good reasons for them, usually of a legal nature.

How, you may ask, is the busy writer or editor to know instantly whether a particular pharmaceutical is a proprietary or a nonproprietary? There are many ways—for one, the United States Pharmacopeial Convention. Its publication of record, which is updated each year, contains the United States Adopted Names (USAN) and current USP (U.S. Pharmacopeia) and NF (National Formulary) names designated for United States nonproprietary drugs and certain chemicals (stains, reagents). It also lists more than 5,000 international nonproprietary names and many proprietary names as well. This work will even tell you how to pronounce the names of generic drugs.

This national treasure, titled *USAN and the USP Dictionary of Drug Names*, can be obtained at some U.S. Government Printing Office stores and certainly from the USPC Order Processing Department 528, 12601 Twinbrook Parkway, Rockville, MD 20852 (toll-free phone, 800-227-USPC). No self-respecting owner of a library for medical editors and writers should be without this authoritative volume.

The *Merck Index* (not to be confused with the *Merck Manual*, a therapeutic guide also indispensable to anyone in the medical field) contains short monographs, descriptions of the "most important chemicals, drugs, pesticides and biologically active substances known" in the United States.

This monumental work, which has been published continuously for 100 years (the first edition was copyrighted in 1889), has been brought up to date only every 8 or 10 years. One look at it will explain why.

Each monograph (entry) includes the cross-indexed common, chemical, or generic name; the chemical formula; the trademark name, if any; and the manufacturer's name. It also includes the year the patent was granted and to whom, as well as other highly pertinent and valuable information such as the supporting documentation, with the names of the initial authors and the journals in which these articles appeared.

Other information in the *Merck Index* includes sections on organic name reactions, radioactive isotopes, isotonic solutions, the International System of Units, universal conversion factors, conversion tables, and Chemical Abstracts names and registry numbers.

The words for the *Merck Index* are *priceless, indispensable,* and *endlessly fascinating.* If ever there was a treasure trove in the form of a textbook, this is it.

Two principal sources for proprietary names are the *American Drug Index* and the *Physicians' Desk Reference,* which are published annually. There are countless others, many of them readily available for reference on the shelves of your medical library or in its computer files through MEDLINE or other authoritative sources.

The *PDR* includes extremely detailed material, most of it taken bodily from the manufacturers' package inserts, about currently used preparations. Note that the *PDR* contains information only about the products or drugs their manufacturers choose to include in the volume that year.

Q.V.

This abbreviation stands for *quod vide,* the Latin for "which see," a suggestion that the reader look up the mentioned term:

> This week's infectious disease report includes a listing for AIDS (q.v.).

The interested reader will take the trouble to find that entry also.

SMITHSONIAN INSTITUTION

The name is *Smithsonian Institution,* not the Smithsonian Institute.

The Smithsonian Institution was founded in 1846 in accordance with the will of James Smithson, a renowned British chemist and mineralogist, who bequeathed his fortune to the United States to create an establishment for the "increase and diffusion of knowledge among men."

It began as a museum. It is now a tremendous complex comprising the National Museum of Natural History, National Museum of History and Technology, National Air and Space Museum, National Zoological Park, Freer Gallery of Art, National Gallery of Art, National Collection of Fine Arts, National Portrait Gallery, Joseph H. Hirshhorn Museum and Sculpture Garden, John F. Kennedy Center for the Performing Arts, Smithsonian Astrophysical Observatory, Smithsonian Tropical Research Institute, Radiation Biology Laboratory, National Armed Forces Museum Advisory Board, Woodrow Wilson International Center for Scholars, Anacostia Neighborhood Museum, National Museum of Design (formerly the Cooper-Hewitt Museum of Decorative Arts and Design), International Exchange Service, and the Science Information Exchange.

TITLES OF JOURNALS AND BOOKS

In medical writing and editing, the titles of journals and books are italicized (underlined in typing). Follow the house style of the journal you're submitting to. If you're uncertain, while you're writing the article, which journal that will be, use the house style of a well-edited journal; chances are you'll be 88 percent in conformity with the publication that will consider your manuscript.

In lists of references in medical works, use *library style* (sometimes called *sentence style*) for titles of articles: initial caps only for the first word and, of course, for proper names and adjectives. Use initial caps (capital letters) and lowercase for titles of books and journals; italicize or use boldface for whichever items are italicized or "bolded" in the journal. (See also "Capitalization in Headings.")

Follow the *Index Medicus* style in general for all items; however, note that *IM* uses not only volume numbers of journals but also issue numbers for the convenience of library users. Using the issue numbers of journals as well as the volume numbers is necessary only when the cited journal does not have consecutive pagination—that is, when each issue starts with page 1. Almost all medical journals use consecutive pagination; each issue picks up from the last page number of the previous issue in any one volume number. In usual practice, each year starts a new volume, so that the first issue of the year begins with page 1.

One-word titles of journals are never abbreviated in lists of references: *Pediatrics*, but *Pediatr Res* (for *Pediatric Research*); *Urology*, but *J Urol* (for *Journal of Urology*). Follow the *Index Medicus* style with respect to abbreviations of journal titles; they are invariable until officially changed by *IM*. Copies of the annual *List of Journals Indexed in Index Medicus* (fondly known as "JIM") can be obtained from the U.S. Government Printing Office.

IM does not use commas, nor does it use periods after initials, within names of authors or after abbreviations in journal titles. Almost all medical journals in the United States follow the *IM* style, with their own modifications for convenience.

TRADEMARKED NAMES

Like the pharmaceutical houses, other manufacturers are anxious to have medical writers and editors observe the rule about capitalizing the first letter of a trademarked name. Certainly the conscientious medical writer or editor will make a sincere effort to ascertain whether a particular name is trademarked. Dictionaries of the English language contain many of these names; stylebooks and libel manuals of the Associated Press and the *New York Times* are also helpful, but only in this respect. These organizations have their own house styles, usually different from medical and pharmaceutical usage.

Among the products that should always be initial-capped are the following:

Band-Aid	Pentothal
Ben-Gay	Plexiglas
Benzedrine	Pyrex
Coca-Cola (and Coke)	Q-Tips
Dexedrine	Scotch tape
Jell-O	Spackle
Kleenex	Styrofoam
Kodak	Technicolor
Masonite	Teflon
Merthiolate	Vaseline
Nembutal	Xerox

If you do use lowercase for one of these names, don't be surprised if you get a letter of gentle complaint from the manufacturer.

Names that have passed into the public domain may be lowercase:

aspirin	lanolin
cellophane	milk of magnesia
dacron	nylon
escalator	orlon
fiberglas(s)	zipper

VESTIGIAL TAILS

Question: Why do some writers and editors (all of impeccable reputation) use -ic and others use -ical in such words as *empiric*, *epidemiologic*, *etiologic*, *pathologic*, *physiologic*, *pharmacologic*, and *psychologic*? My practice is to omit -al when it is unnecessary, that is, when either version would be correct. In words of this kind, nothing is lost if the tail is removed, and nothing is gained if the tail is added. The meaning is the same.

However, there are some words that have different meanings, depending on whether the -al tail is used. *Classic* and *classical* and *historic* and *historical* come instantly to mind. *Physic* and *physical* are another pair.

The 1989 AMA *Manual of Style* says that "in most scientific writing, the adjective *classic* generally means 'authentic,' 'authoritative,' or 'typical' (the *classic* symptoms of myocardial infarction include chest pain, nausea, and diaphoresis). In contrast, *classical* has to do with the humanities or the fine arts (a *classical* column, unlike a medieval column or pier, is strictly defined and self-sufficient)."

Webster III, in its usage notes under *classic*, was probably referring to Linnaeus (real name, Carl von Linné), the Swedish botanist who established a system of binomial nomenclature, as the author of a "manual of botany [that] has become a *classic* among scientists." A *classical* scholar is one devoted to the literature or languages of ancient Greece and Rome. Many members of the clergy (of whatever faith or denomination) are classical scholars.

Wilson Follett wrote in *Modern American Usage* that events holding an important place in history are *historic*. "Thus Napoleon's return from Elba was a *historic* event, President Monroe's doctrine of 1823 a *historic* utterance."

This mnemonic association may help to fix the nuances in your mind:

hi*stor*ic	*s*pecial *story*
histori*cal*	actu*al*

What is important or famous in history or that which is making history is *historic*. That which is about history or based on history is *historical*.

In words such as *logic* and *logical*, there's no contest. There is a definite difference. *Logic* is a noun and *logical* is an adjective; it is unlikely that there would be confusion. Although *politic* and *political* are both adjectives, they have different meanings; what is political is not always *politic* (expedient or judicious). The adjectives *fanatic* and *hysteric* have themselves become nouns, so that the *-al* tail is used when the adjectival form is needed.

In writing and editing, the shorter and unambiguous term is preferable if the house style does not preclude its use. And thus ends the tale.

VIRGULE AND PER

Don't use the virgule (/) and don't abbreviate in terms without numbers; use *per* instead:

Values are expressed in milligrams per deciliter.

One such measure is respirations per minute.

The dosage was adjusted, in accordance with the protocol, to a certain number of milligrams per kilogram of body weight per day.

The patient's cardiac output was estimated to be 5 to 6 L/min on the basis of 70 heartbeats per minute and a stroke volume of 80 mL.

VON

In reading and citing articles in German, remember that *von* is not only part of some German names—it also means "by," as in "written by." If the *von* on the article's title page is on a line by itself, you can be certain that it means "written by." If you see *von* in a list of references, make sure that it is indeed part of an author's name by referring to the title page of the original article.

This error points up the hazard of using secondary references—those you've borrowed from other authors' lists of references—rather than the original articles. I have learned from painful experience never to trust second-hand or filtered-down references, and I therefore insist on having in hand photocopies of cited articles before I edit a work. This practice ultimately saves innumerable hours. As the cynical saying goes, "There's never enough time to do things right in the first place, but there's always time to do them over"—and over and over.

As I've discussed elsewhere, studies by respected editors and others show that half to three quarters of all references in lists of references contain at least one inaccurate item.

YAG

YAG, as in YAG laser surgery, for example, is an abbreviation for yttrium-aluminum-garnet.

ZIP CODE

The official two-letter ZIP code designations (without periods) for the names of states should be used only when a ZIP code number actually follows the state's name. In all other contexts, spell out the name or use the traditional state abbreviation:

> National Library of Medicine, 8600 Rockville Pike, Bethesda, MD 20894
>
> The National Institutes of Health complex is located in Bethesda, Maryland (or Md.).
>
> His mentor resides in Palo Alto, Calif.

I find it annoying to have to guess whether MN means Maine or Minnesota (it means the latter). Some astute organizations use both the conventional abbreviation (Fla., Pa., N.Y.) and the two-letter state designation (FL, PA, NY) on their letterheads for, I hope, precisely this reason.

The names of some states are never abbreviated in text unless followed by a ZIP code: Texas, Ohio, Idaho, Iowa, Alaska, Hawaii.

The acronym ZIP, as in ZIP code, stands for *zone improvement program* or *plan*. Some publishers or others who aren't aware of what it stood for in the first place print it as *zip* or *Zip*.

CHAPTER 5

Grammar and Usage

Although it might seem that *bad grammar* is a contradiction in terms—a seeming oxymoron—this term is correct. So is *grammatical error*, a term in which the adjective means not "an error that is correct grammatically"—an illogical concept—but merely "pertaining to grammar." For the same reason, *moral turpitude* is correct; however, this oxymoron, which comes trippingly to the tongues of Bowdlerians and Comstockians, seems redundant to me.

There are splendid books on English grammar and usage, which should be consulted for details of principles and practice.

Victor Hugo wrote (perhaps sadly, perhaps cynically) that everything bows to success—even grammar.

In this chapter I discuss some common grammatical and usage errors in medical writing. Naturally, the topics will overlap with those of other chapters, and therefore some repetition is inevitable. Reinforcement is a powerful mnemonic tool.

ABSTRACTIONS AND PLURALS

Should one have tolerance and other people have tolerances?

Is it preferable to continue one's education and for others to continue their educations?

It might seem logical to use the plural if there is more than one person referred to. The idiomatic usage, however, is to use the singular, even when several persons or things are mentioned, if the noun is an attribute possessed in common or is an abstraction. Curiosity killed the cat; three cats do not have three curiosities—they all have curiosity.

To get back to *tolerance* and *tolerances*:

> The preamble to the United Nations charter said that the organization was formed "to practice tolerance and live together in peace with one another as good neighbors."
>
> The mints deal with extremely small tolerances in making coins.

The question will arise as to whether *behavior* and other such words (abstractions) can be used in the plural. One school (of which I am a member) says that behavior is behavior, and that there can be only *kinds of* behavior if the plural is needed; that arrhythmia is arrhythmia, and that there can be many *types of* arrhythmia. Another school asserts stoutly that *arrhythmia* can be used in the plural, and indeed *arrhythmias* is firmly entrenched in medical terminology. *Behaviors* is equally firmly entrenched in psychologic and psychiatric terminology. This point may constitute a *lost cause* (*L.C.*). Authors will probably continue to use these plurals no matter what I prefer.

ACTIVE VS. PASSIVE VOICE

In the past, reports of research were almost always written in the passive voice. This was *de rigueur*. So was pedantic, pedestrian, dry-as-dust writing.

Things have changed. Today the editors of medical journals and books encourage the active voice, as they should. If the investigation merited the work entailed in writing a report, surely the report itself should not be weasel-worded. The authors should be proud to say, "We performed the requisite studies," rather than "The requisite studies were performed" . . . if indeed they *had* done the studies.

The active voice places the responsibility for the design of the study, the protocol, the methods, and the conclusions squarely where it belongs—on the shoulders of the investigators and ultimately the author or authors. Use of the active voice may even disinhibit the authors enough to make the work bloodful rather than bloodless.

It is not "more scientific" and "objective" to use the passive voice; it is only more imprecise—and cowardly. However, circumstances sometimes necessitate use of the passive voice to avoid absurdities or convoluted phraseology. Here, as everywhere and always, good sense and judgment—hallmarks of the good editor—will prevail and will suggest the choice. If it is not really important to know which specific unit did the laboratory studies, for example, the passive voice is appropriate.

Instead of writing "This article reports the results . . ." or "In this article are reported the results . . .," the authors of the example given below used the straightforward active voice:

In this article, we report the results of a time-trend, case-control study of a population of individuals who sought periodic comprehensive medical examinations.

Here are other examples of good use of the active voice:

We conducted a series of life-table analyses.

To ensure equivalency, to the degree possible, of subjects' baseline status, we required all of them to be free of middle-ear effusion at their trial starting point.

Examples of good use of the passive voice:

To determine the relation between serum cholesterol level and the development of colon cancer, a case-control study was designed.

The children whose parents withheld consent were enrolled in a separate, nonrandomized but otherwise identical trial and were assigned according to parental preference.

As part of their monitoring, most subjects were tested audiometrically during and after episodes of otitis media.

Using the active voice may even make a scientific paper or book more lively as well as informative. It is possible to write factually *and* interestingly. The pity is that it is so seldom done, sometimes because of an unwarranted fear that the reader will think less of the author, her or his scientific objectivity, or the work if the manuscript is interesting.

Professor Richard Mitchell, of Glassboro (New Jersey) State College, an eminent grammarian and author, wrote that in using the passive voice, the "writer is putting as much distance as possible between himself and what he says. . . . People who write like that are in flight from the responsibility implied by the basic structure of the English in which doers do deeds."

AND OR OR

Sometimes the use of *and* instead of *or* produces an absurdity:

Three patients died during and after coronary bypass surgery.

Three patients died twice? Of course not:

Three patients died during *or* after coronary bypass surgery.

AS BEST AS

It is incorrect to say, "She solved the problem as best as she could."

In the correct sentence "She solved the problem as best she could," *as* indicates the way or the manner. *As* . . . *as* indicates degree. Similarly, it would be incorrect to say, "as richest as Croesus." *Best* already indicates the degree as a superlative, that is, the highest degree. These sentences too would be correct:

> She solved the problem as well as she could.
> She solved the problem the best way she could.

AS GOOD AS

> From the data, the investigators determined that in these particular cases radiation and chemotherapy were as good or better than radical surgery.

"As good *as* or better than" would be the proper wording. In conversation it's easy to forget that there is another *as* coming; in writing it is inexcusable.

BETWEEN THE CRACKS

> Millions of children and their parents living just above the poverty line fall between the Medicaid cracks.

Since it is physically impossible for anything to fall *between* cracks (which are empty spaces, after all), the proper prepositional phrase is *through the cracks.*

BLAME ON

> The medical officer blamed the deaths on an unnamed tropical parasite.

The wrong thing is being blamed. The deaths were not responsible for the parasite—the parasite was responsible for the deaths:

> The medical officer blamed an unnamed tropical parasite for the deaths.

COMPARE TO, WITH

When two or more things are being compared for similarities *and* dissimilarities, use *compare with.* When you want to liken two things or persons, use *compare to. Compare with* is almost always correct. *Compare to* almost always has a figurative implication.

> It was like comparing apples with oranges.
> Shall I compare thee to a summer's day?
> It is futile to compare the economy of an underdeveloped country with that of an industrial nation.

Many scholars would compare Learned Hand to Oliver Wendell Holmes.

DANGLING MODIFIERS

Due to the volume of other articles submitted this month, we have postponed the symposium on arrhythmia.

We are due to the volume of articles? No, no. The sentence could be changed to read "Because of the volume . . ."

Some grammarians sanction *due to* even when it does not modify anything, because they consider it an absolute adverbial phrase. The stricter authorities still consider *due* an adjective and therefore necessarily the modifier of a noun.

Due to can also mean "caused by":

Their death was due to pneumonia.

I don't use *due to* unless it modifies a noun; I sometimes substitute *because of,* if that is what is meant:

Their flight to the West for the colloqium was postponed because of (not due to) a severe windstorm.

Owing to can almost always be substituted for *due to,* especially at the beginning of a sentence.

Because it is a time-saver, the incorrect use of *due to* has gained acceptance by lazy writers as a handy phrase to be used anywhere in a sentence, that is, without regard to its grammatical appropriateness.

It is almost a certainty that *due to* correctly used only as an adjective phrase is an L.C.

There are other kinds of dangling modifiers. These absolute constructions should—like good medicine—be used with caution. The writer must be sure that the absolute is not modifying the subject of the sentence:

A lifelong Mormon, her ancestors became church members soon after its founding.

Her ancestors were a lifelong Mormon? Apparently the writer meant that the *she* of "her" ancestors was a lifelong Mormon.

Built in 1765, the first mayor of Philadelphia lived here.

Take my word for it: The first mayor of Philadelphia was not built in 1765.

Based on these experiments, we concluded that the acetone-extractable lipids were a requirement for enzymatic activity.

The job of the writer is to make facts and ideas *instantly* intelligible. No reader should have to read a sentence twice or three times to figure out that "we" are not "based on these experiments." A simple way out of that paper bag is to use "on the basis of these experiments."

Dangling modifiers should be differentiated from absolute constructions. *Absolute constructions* are so called because they are grammatically independent of anything else in the sentence and do not always have a subject. They are idiomatic and are not meant or expected to modify anything in the sentence. The *absolute* part comes from the Latin *absolutus*, the past participle of *absolvere*, to "set free" or "absolve."

The following are some examples of absolute constructions and participles that are stock phrases or absolutes. Sometimes these words and phrases appear in the middle or end of a sentence, but they usually stand at the head:

according to	granted
conceivably	in regard to
concerning	judging from (or by)
considering the facts (or cir-	more important(ly)
cumstances)	provided
generally speaking	regarding
getting down to brass tacks	speaking of
given the facts (or circum-	
stances)	

Here again, the writer must think ahead to the subject of the sentence to make sure that the absolute is not modifying it, especially with such phrases as *judging from* and *given (or considering) the facts*:

Judging from the facts, the attorney was prudent enough to continue the case.

Did the attorney judge from the facts or is *judging* an absolute in this context? The sentence is ambiguous; this opening participial phrase can be classified as either a dangling modifier or an absolute construction. The writer must be queried.

DIFFERENT FROM, DIFFERENT THAN

Why writers write *different than* when they wouldn't write *differ than* is beyond me. Here is an incorrect usage:

The malpractice and "good Samaritan" laws in New York differ than those in Pennsylvania.

Differ from is undoubtedly correct, in all instances.
So is *different from*:

Wherein is cardiac disease different from cardiovascular disease?

Except in one circumstance, *different* is *not* the comparative form of an adjective; therefore, it should not be followed by *than*. One would not say "good than," but one could say "better [comparative] than." In the following sentence, *different* becomes a comparative:

Fraternal twins are more different [from each other] than identical twins [are different from each other].

If *different from* would create an impossible, convoluted sentence, most usage experts (Wilson Follett vigorously dissenting) agree that *different than* is preferable. Follett preferred to recast the sentence to clarify; he wrote that *differently than* is not preferred, since the *differently than* can almost always be replaced by *otherwise than*.

In short, the consensus is that *different from* is always right, especially in a straightforward sentence, but that *different than* may be used if a complicated clause follows.

Good editors will always change *different than* to *different from* in a straightforward sentence; they will also be happy to recast a tortuous sentence if that becomes necessary.

DISAGREEMENT IN NUMBER OF VERB

Consumption of large amounts of sugar cause an inflated level of insulin.

The writer didn't keep her or his eye on the ball. The verb should be *causes,* since the subject of the sentence is the singular *consumption,* not the plural *amounts.*

The growing complexity and technical requirements of nuclear imaging equipment is the price paid for the satisfactory results obtained.

The verb should be the plural *are,* since there is more than one subject: *complexity* and *requirements.* The subject rules the number of the verb, no matter how far it is from the verb.

DISSIMILAR

Oddly enough, the adjective *dissimilar* takes the preposition *to,* just as its antonym, *similar,* does:

Opioids are dissimilar to opiates in certain pharmacokinetic aspects.

The error of using *dissimilar from* probably arises from the knowledge that *dissimilar* means "different."

Webster III has it both ways in its usage examples.

DRUG, DRAGGED

Despite its common use in certain regions of the United States, *drug* is substandard in serious writing as the past tense of *drag*, which is *dragged*. This characterization does not apply to fiction or dialogue in writing.

A popular character on television, an Atlanta attorney, uses this dialectical word deliberately to foster the local impression that he is only a "good ole country boy," although he is as sophisticated and literate as any Philadelphia lawyer.

ENSURE, INSURE

Dictionaries list them as synonyms, but I prefer to use *ensure* to mean assure, guarantee, or make certain, and to limit *insure* to the realm of life, home, flight, or auto insurance.

Ensure is from the Middle English *ensuren*, which is from the Anglo-French *enseuren*. *Insure* is from ME *insuren*. Both are probably ultimately from Old French *aseurer*, "to assure."

> A strict policy on sterility ensures the safety of the patient.
>
> The institution is to assume the cost of insuring the staff against malpractice.

The word *ensurance* is obsolete; the noun for both kinds of assurance is *insurance*.

EQUALLY AS

Equally as is redundant and always incorrect.

> The cardiac output is equally as important.

Delete either *equally* or *as*.

A person can be *as alert as* another or *equally alert*. What she or he cannot be is "equally as" alert.

FEWER, LESS

Good writing and editing call for differentiation between *fewer*, which is used for number, and *less*, which is used for quantity or, sometimes, abstractions:

> Fewer deaths caused by infectious diseases are now being recorded than at any other time in history.
>
> There is less danger of error with a biostatistician on the protocol designing team.

FIT, FITTED

The past tense of *fit* is *fitted*, despite some dictionaries. The past tense of *outfit* is *outfitted* and of *befit, befitted.*

The past tense of *bet* is *betted.*

See also "Pit, Pitted."

FLY

The past tense of *fly* is not always *flew.*

In his last at-bat, he flied out.

Watch those flying typos!

I, WE

Just as medical writers should use the active voice rather than the passive most of the time, the author of a report should use *I* along with the active voice. Out of mistaken modesty, some solo investigators use *we* rather than *I*. The sole investigator, or the sole writer, should take full responsibility for her or his work by using *I* instead of hiding behind an amorphous *we*.

Some researchers fear that they will be accused of lack of objectivity if they use the active voice and *I* or *we*. On the contrary, professional credibility is tarnished when writers use the passive voice and keep the reader in the dark as to who actually did the work. The reader should know who is responsible for the report's factual, grammatical, and medical accuracy, not to mention its integrity.

When I use *I* rather than *we*, it is not out of arrogance or egotism but rather out of an honest desire to be accountable for my own mistakes. *We* should be reserved for royalty ("We are not amused"), legitimate editorial, and other appropriate uses.

The modern move from the traditional obligatory *we* to *I* is an improvement. Most of the prestigious and the best edited—not always interchangeable terms—journals prefer that authors use *I* for a lone author as well as the active voice, and so request in their instructions. In *Modern American Usage*, Wilson Follett wrote:

> Resolve to take the great leap and say *I*. Everybody should by now recognize that a mask is more conspicuous than a face.

IF, WHETHER

These two words can often be used interchangeably, but there are exceptions, depending on the meaning. If *if* renders the sentence ambiguous, don't use it.

> The graduates wanted to know if they were going to be matched by computer for residencies.

Does that mean *whenever* they were going to be matched or *whether* they would be matched by computers or by humans?

Use either *if* or *whether* unless the meaning could be misconstrued. *If* suggests a condition; *whether* usually implies an alternative or doubt.

Whether, being unambiguous, is correct in almost all instances.

IN, INTO

Don't be offended if someone tells you to jump *in* the lake; the sports director is merely recommending more strenuous activity than floating or dog-paddling. Do be offended if someone tells you to jump *into* the lake.

These two prepositions are often used interchangeably, but there is a difference. *Into* denotes *in*, but with an addendum: direction or motion. In the first instance, the subject is already *in* the water; in the second, *out* of the water but moving toward it.

There is a further delicate differentiation:

> Look in the textbook for clarification.
> Look into the commission's report immediately.

The first instance suggests reading the textbook; the second strongly recommends a thorough examination of the report, with a view to learning much more about it.

LAY, LIE

These two verbs cause more confusion and trouble than almost any other words in the English language. One way to keep them straight and thus mark oneself as an educated, cultured person is to remember that one of these verbs always takes an object; the other, never.

The principal parts of *lie* are lie, lay, lain, lying. It is an intransitive verb (never takes an object) and is usually followed by *down*.

The principal parts of *lay* are lay, laid, laid, laying. It is a transitive verb (almost always takes an object).

> The remedy lies in education.
> The patient lay on the bed while doing passive exercises.

On the advice of his physician, he has always lain down for an afternoon nap.

The books were lying open to keep the backs from breaking.

I always lay my manuals on the computer table.

He laid his cause before the high commissioner.

They have laid their burdens on this department far too long.

Laying bricks and stones is an ancient occupation; one thinks of the pyramids of Egypt.

LIGATURES

Sutures are not the only ligatures. *Ligature,* from the Latin *ligere,* to bind or tie, is used in music, printing, musical instrumentation, witchcraft, and magic.

In editorial notation, ligatures are curved lines (like parentheses turned on their sides), used with a slash to indicate that a seemingly hyphenated word is actually solid.

In printing, a ligature is a character consisting of two or more letters combined into one: æ, œ, ff, fl, ffl, and so on. Today such physically combined letters are seen less and less; double vowels such as *ae* and *oe* are used more commonly. The word processor has had some influence here.

In British usage the ligatures, or double vowels, *oe* and *ae* are seen in such words as *foetus* and *orthopaedics.* American usage has simplified these ligatures or double vowels in most words to a simple *e,* since the pronunciation is the same whether *oe* or *ae* is used or just *e.*

Some associations and disciplines insist on the double vowel (but rarely the ligature) in such words as *aegis, aesthetics, aestivation, anaesthesiology, haemostasis, mediaeval, oenanthic, oenology, orthopaedics,* and *paediatrics.* However, in ordinary usage the simple *e* is used rather than *oe* or *ae* in words that were formerly written with the double vowel or ligature, such as *asafoetida, oecumenical* (Late Latin, and ultimately from the Greek *oikoumenos,* inhabited, from *oikos,* house or habitation), *oenocyte, oesophagus, oestrogen, oestrus, paedagogy* (from the Greek *pais,* child, and *agogos,* leader or teacher), and *poenology* (from the Greek *poine,* penalty).

A word of caution: Consistency is the watchword. If the ligature or double vowel is used once in a work, it should be used throughout the work. American editors should not presume to edit British-style works unless they are thoroughly conversant with British usage and spelling—not only as to ligatures or double vowels but also as to the *ou* (as in *labour*) usage and other ramifications. British spelling and usage contain many pitfalls for the unwary American writer or editor.

Taxonomic terms, such as the names of bacteria and other microorganisms, are *invariable* and are *never simplified or altered.* The double vowel, if any, is *always* used. Consult *Bergey's Manual* (see Buchanan and Gibbons in the Bibliography for the full citation) for the names, plural forms, italicization, and other rules with regard to bacteria and other organisms. (See also "Bacteria," in Chapter 4.)

Certain names, such as Caesar, Aeschylus, and Oedipus, always retain the double vowel but are not printed or typed with the two combined into one.

ONE WHO

A common error is the use of a singular verb after "one of those who" or similar constructions:

> The researcher is not one of those who is willing to compromise his principles.

It should read "one of those who are willing." The clause beginning with *who* modifies *those,* not *one,* and so a plural verb should be used to conform with the plural those.

OTHER

A common error is to omit *other* in categorizing:

> A reduced version of George Gershwin's *Rhapsody in Blue* will be performed as well as selected works of American composers.

That should read "*other* American composers"; otherwise, it could be mistakenly assumed that Gershwin is not an American composer.

> Psychiatrists are better equipped to deal with depression than most physicians.

Most *other* physicians. As the grammatically inadequate writer probably knew, psychiatrists *are* physicians.

PARALLELISM

Lack of parallelism is the cause of many common errors, particularly in journalism, where deadlines rule and carefulness is not always possible.

> This famous editor-writer from a New York university does not hesitate to chastise medical writers who already have or are likely to bypass his recommendations.

This should read "who already have bypassed or are likely to bypass his recommendations."

The medical profession has not and will not shirk this responsibility.

The first verb in that sentence should be "has not *shirked*," since otherwise it would read "The medical profession has not shirk this responsibility," a grammatical monstrosity.

> The police officer resigned after he was arrested on charges of being drunk, disorderly and firing his gun into the air after questioning the students.

This sentence should be reworded, since otherwise it would read "on charges of being firing." An *and* between drunk and disorderly would repair the sentence:

> The police officer resigned after he was arrested on charges of being drunk and disorderly and firing his gun into the air after questioning the students.

The incorrect version of the sentence is an example of the "slovenliness" castigated by Fowler (as cited in Nicholson's *A Dictionary of American-English Usage*, which is based on Fowler's *Modern English Usage*). In a masterly coinage, which has survived the passage of several decades, he called this lack of parallelism a "bastard enumeration": "There is perhaps no blunder by which hasty writing is so commonly defaced [as the one cited]."

> You'll save money, energy and keep warm.

Another bastard enumeration. What's needed is another *and* between *money* and *energy*. In this compound sentence, one can easily see that "You'll save money, energy" is incorrect. Each clause should be able to stand independently:

> You'll save money and energy and [you'll] keep warm.

The following sentence has the proper number of *and*s:

> As designed, the clinic building will be multilevel and multifaceted and have copper trimming.

Some phrases are left incomplete:

> The new style of leadership is characterized by an unobtrusive femininity that works as well, or better, than traditional male leadership styles.

"That works *as* well *as*, or better than, traditional male leadership styles." Another way to recast this controversial statement is to write "that works as well as traditional male leadership styles, or better."

> Declaring oneself a candidate too soon can be as self-defeating, or more so, than a long-delayed announcement.

"*As* self-defeating *as* a long-delayed announcement, or more so." Lack of parallelism is the fault in these examples:

> Healthier living through modifications in life style: reduction of weight, salt intake, smoking, stress, anxieties and proper programs of exercise, rest and relaxation.

"Reduction of proper programs"? No. The following is a better way to put this verbless but not telegraphic recommendation:

> Healthier living through modifications in life style: reduction of weight, salt intake, smoking, stress, and anxieties, and initiation of proper programs of exercise, rest, and relaxation.

Here's another complicated sentence:

> Studies with this drug have confirmed its therapeutic value for healing, relief of pain, and epigastric discomfort in certain patients.

Studies have confirmed its value for epigastric discomfort? The writer certainly did not intend to say that. The thought can be clarified by placing *and* after *healing; and for* would be even better:

> Studies with this drug have confirmed its therapeutic value for healing and for relief of pain and epigastric discomfort in certain patients.

Another kind of lack of parallelism is the change of verb number in midstream:

> A large quantity of arms and ammunition was seized and about 150 hostages freed.

This should have read "A large quantity of arms and ammunition *was* seized and about 150 hostages *were* freed."

PIT, PITTED

The past tense of *pit* is *pitted.* Proper use of the past tense obviates ambiguity; the reader doesn't have to wonder whether the action is taking place or whether it took place in the past:

> The young pit their strength against the power of the establishment.

Does that mean that the young *always* pit their strength against the establishment or that the young *pitted* their strength in the past? The sociologist who wrote that sentence should be queried.

PREPOSITION AT END OF SENTENCE

There is no reason for the "rule" that a preposition is not something you end a sentence with. People who insist on this dogma don't know what they're talking about. One often wonders what other mischief they're up to.

The following sentences are grammatically correct:

> Put up or shut up.
> I question what those regulations are for.
> What's it all about?
> Those restrictions should be done away with.

As was so often the case, Winston Churchill had the last word. This quotation is attributed to him:

> This is the sort of English up with which I will not put.

I've also heard it quoted as:

> This is the sort of arrant pedantry up with which I will not put.

Although Wolcott Gibbs was thinking of the *Time-Life-Fortune* mode of writing rather than of Churchill's retort, he wrote:

> Backward ran sentences until reeled the mind. . . . Where it will all end, knows God!

PROVED, PROVEN

Proved is the past tense of *prove*. The past participle *proven* is obsolete as the past tense; however, it is sometimes used as an adjective to precede a noun:

> Both sides have proved their cases over and over.
> Their method is an accepted, proven technique.

SINCE, BECAUSE

There is a common misconception that *since* is always temporal, that is, having only to do with time, and therefore it should not be used to mean *because*. *Since* was used as a causal conjunction introducing an adverbial clause even before Chaucer; it goes back to Old English *sithence* (*sith-than*), meaning "after that." Later it took on the figurative meaning of "given that" or "because."

Since and *because* are synonymous when they're used as causal conjunctions. To avoid ambiguity, use a comma before *since* when it introduces a nonrestrictive causal clause. Don't use a comma when it introduces a restrictive temporal clause, that is, one that describes the timing of the main verb:

> Nouns have been used as adjectives to modify other nouns since the English language has existed [temporal, restrictive adverbial clause].
>
> The candidate spoke in Spanish, since he wished to please the town's inhabitants [causal, nonrestrictive adverbial clause].

Since can also be used as an adverb or a preposition:

> She has since become an officer of the corporation [adverb].
>
> The department head has been away from his desk since noon [preposition].

Many of us writers alternate our causal clauses with *since* and *because* for the sake of variety.

SINGULAR OR PLURAL VERB?

Should the singular or the plural verb be used in these examples?

> A number of patients (was)(were) selected for the investigation.
>
> A total of 257 products (was)(were) designated as orphan drugs by the FDA; 33 have been approved for marketing.
>
> The number of erythrocytes (was)(were) excessive.
>
> The total of students who were living on campus (was)(were) above capacity.

A number (*a* total) takes a plural verb. *The* number (*the* total) takes a singular verb.

When *none* means not any, a plural verb is preferable:

> None of the institutions in the consortium have solutions to the problem of the uninsured.

When *none* specifically means not one, a singular verb is preferable:

> As to the candidates for postdoctoral fellowships, none is from this geographic area.

In sentences with more than one subject, the linkage *neither . . . nor* may raise a question as to whether a singular or a plural verb should be used:

> Neither the senior nor the junior was in the running for the fellowship. (Both linked nouns are singular.)
>
> Neither the sisters nor the brothers were named heirs. (Both linked nouns are plural.)

If the two or more linked nouns are singular *and* plural, the noun nearer or nearest the verb gets to call the tune:

Neither the vice presidents nor the chief operating officer was a member of the other board.

Neither the pediatrician nor the nurses were able to tell the twins apart at first glance.

A singular verb is often mistakenly used when a plural one is called for in sentences containing *one of the*:

Rogers Bioengineering is one of the few companies in the world that covers the whole range of diagnostic imaging and treatment systems.

The verb should be *cover,* since it refers back to the subject *companies,* not the spurious subject *Rogers Bioengineering.* If the sentence is turned around, the point is made clear:

Of the few companies in the world that cover the whole range of diagnostic imaging and treatment systems, Rogers Bioengineering is one.

SPLIT INFINITIVES

The prohibition against split infinitives has endured an astoundingly long time. Although writers should not go out of their way to split infinitives, they should not agonize over them when the infinitives beg for splitting. How else could one express these thoughts without awkwardness?

Slightly built football players are sometimes able *to more than hold* their own against larger rivals.

For many years researchers have been attempting *to genetically alter* certain viruses.

The agreement compelled the administration *to more than double* the director's salary.

The profession has begun *to not only acknowledge* that more than laws are needed, but to flesh out its belief that solutions must be sought in the community.

Bernstein said many years ago, "the taboo seems to really be on the way out." I believe it is now kaput, obsolete, extinct, fini. And good riddance!

There are situations in which splitting becomes mandatory:

Her main objective was to be properly educated.

In this example, putting *properly* after *educated* would change the meaning—subtly but inaccurately.

Some time ago a reader asked me, with tongue planted firmly in cheek, whether it is true that split infinitives are the first step to moral decay. I responded that his question was of such profound significance that I would consult an expert on morals *and* on split infinitives. Not having found one, I was constrained to reply as a person who had had much to do with grammar but very little to do with morals.

After much research and contemplation, I reported my findings. However, since my study population was so small, my findings require validation by other investigators: Of a total of 10 users of split infinitives, I found one to be the head of a terrorist group; one had become the head of a money-laundering empire; and one had been an unindicted co-conspirator in the Watergate *cause célèbre.* Evidence showed that the remaining seven subjects were upright citizens who had never been in trouble with the law, except for one who had been charged with abusing a brainchild but had never been convicted.

On the basis of these findings, I concluded that six or seven out of ten isn't bad and that splitting infinitives is not an index of moral decay. *There is nothing wrong morally or grammatically with splitting infinitives.*

As Wilson Follett so musically stated, "Like parallel fifths in harmony, the split infinitive is the one fault that everybody has heard about and makes a great virtue of avoiding and reproving in others. . . . Shaw had delivered the controlling opinion: 'Every good literary craftsman splits his infinitives when the sense demands it. I call for the immediate dismissal of the pedant on the staff who chases split infinitives. It is of no consequence whether he decides to go quickly or to quickly go.'"

SUBJUNCTIVE

> If there were not one central government, each state would have to issue visas.

The subjunctive in the preceding sentence denotes a condition contrary to fact—there *is* a central government.

> If he were a citizen, he would be eligible to run for president.

This is another condition contrary to fact: The referent *he* is an alien, and so is ineligible.

Many writers have the mistaken notion that *if* should always be followed by a subjunctive verb. Especially in the past tense, *if* can indicate an actual condition or situation:

> If he was in the classroom, he was included in the roll call.

In the following sentences, the subjunctive verb *were* denotes a wish or hypothetical circumstance:

> I wish that I were in New Orleans for Mardi Gras.

UNICEF and WHO say that measles, a main cause of death from disease in children, could be eradicated if every child in the world were inoculated and immunized against it.

If I were king, I'd declare a constitutional monarchy.

Since I am not king (and a good thing too), the subjunctive mood (*were*) is used.

If can introduce a clause of supposition, in which event the indicative (*are*), not the subjunctive (*be*), is used:

If he is [not were] successful in his investigation, the findings will benefit more than a thousand farm workers in Ohio.

The subjunctive is used after verbs denoting a request or an order:

The court ordered that he be deported to his native country.

Grammarians are generally agreed that the subjunctive mood is obsolescent and, in the main, unnecessary. There are exceptions (in addition to the "king" example) in which the subjunctive is obligatory, or almost so: "certain almost ritualistic phrases" (Opdycke, p. 136), quotations, and catchphrases:

If this be treason, make the most of it.
Thy will be done.
Though it be ragged and battle-worn, yet will Old Glory wave forevermore.

In bygone days, Britons and Americans used to say, "If the day be rainy, we shall stay at home." We no longer talk like that. Most people use the indicative mood instead of the subjunctive most of the time because the indicative serves equally well.

Opdycke wrote that "there is no particular advantage to writing 'Even though it hurt me, I will still do it' rather than 'Even though it hurts me, I will still do it.'"

THAT, WHICH

I am extremely careful in my use of *that* and *which* in relative clauses. Interchangeable use or misuse of these relative pronouns can lead to ambiguity and needless confusion.

There are those who see nothing wrong with using *which* interchangeably with *that*. I once was conversing with a student on this very subject, explaining that the misuse of *which* can be ludicrous. He listened to me as I recited part of the nursery rhyme about the house that Jack built, substituting the incorrect *which* for the actual *that* of the rhyme: ". . . which ate the malt which lay in the house which Jack built." All he said was, "What's your point?" I gave up.

If you listen carefully to non-English speakers on television, you'll notice that they rarely use the defining relative pronoun *that* even when it would be correct. I can almost always discern a nonnative speaker from the numerous *which* (nondefining relative pronoun) clues. The bogus *which*-rich excerpt from *Jack* sounds as if it were written by a visiting European.

Which would also be ludicrous in the grammatically correct title of Rudyard Kipling's book *The Light That Failed*. Follett calls the misuse of *which* uncouth, and cites these errors as a "final demonstration of the difference between the natural and the unnatural idiom, and incidentally of the stylistic havoc that can be wrought by very simple means."

Restrictive and nonrestrictive clauses are topics for the grammar and usage textbooks I've mentioned. However, since *that* and *which* figure so prominently in speech and writing, and ambiguities are committed unnecessarily, I decided to discuss these particular words here in their function as relative pronouns introducing such clauses.

Look at this seemingly simple sentence, which turns out to be a subtle exercise in usage and medical information:

> Oral drugs are indicated in the management of diabetes mellitus (which)(that) cannot be treated with diet alone.

In this context, *which* would mean that diabetes mellitus cannot be treated with diet alone—a medically inaccurate statement. The correct choice here is *that*, because in this context it means that this particular form of diabetes can and should be treated with oral drugs if proper diet is inadequate.

Wilson Follett (*Modern American Usage*) and Theodore Bernstein (*The Careful Writer*) devote five and three pages respectively to the differentiation between *that* and *which* as relative pronouns at the head of restrictive (*that*) or nondefining, nonrestrictive (*which*) clauses.

In an opinion handed down in 1928, Supreme Court Justice Oliver Wendell Holmes, Jr. (Holmes *père* was the illustrious physician, philosopher, wit, and writer) wrote these unforgettable words in *United States v. Schwimmer*, 279 U.S. 644, 653:

> If there is any principle of the Constitution that more imperatively calls for attachment than any other, it is the principle of free thought—not free thought for those who agree with us but freedom for the thought that we hate.

That can often be omitted; *which* as a nondefining pronoun cannot.

> The investigation (that) we conducted has been replicated by other researchers.

One way of deciding whether to use *that* or *which*, either in speech or writing, is to see whether the clause in question can be omitted without vitiating the meaning—that is, whether the clause is in effect parenthetical. If it cannot be so omitted, use *that*.

Another empiric method is always to use *that* unless you could justifiably place a comma before the *clause*. The use of *which* mandates a preceding comma.

That should not be used, however, to define an already defined thought or entity. Here is an incorrect use:

> The Food and Drug Administration that promulgated the regulations will hasten the evaluation of these drugs.

The FDA is the only agency that could promulgate these regulations; therefore, the sentence should read:

> The Food and Drug Administration, which promulgated the regulations, will hasten the evaluation of these drugs.

Certainly the two words should never be intermixed for elegant variation.

When a demonstrative *that* and a relative *that* would be juxtaposed, the second one becomes *which*:

> One does that which comes naturally—preferably the right thing.

When the relative follows a preposition, such as *of*, the phrase is always *of which*:

> Alcohol abuse clinics, of which there are fortunately many in this state, are helpful in the treatment of patients who abuse other drugs as well.

The relative *who* refers to persons or people, *which* to things, and *that* to either persons, people, or things.

Because speech is more telegraphic than writing and includes fewer clauses, the uses of *that* will far outnumber those of *which*. In writing, which tends to be more complex and sometimes even circuitous, the uses of *which* are much more numerous than in speech.

Words are instruments to clarify. I believe that the distinction between *that* and *which* is important and should be preserved.

UNDER WAY

In almost all instances, this adverbial term consists of two words, not one.

> The laminectomy was soon under way.

There is an exception to the rule that *under way* must be two words: This term can be used as an adjective meaning occurring, performed, or used while traveling or in motion, in which case it is one word:

> An underway [mobile] emergency unit was quickly dispatched.

WHO, WHOM

> Youm, that's whom.

> Dear Abby: I would like a straight answer. In order for a person to get places in this world, is it what you know or who you know?
>
> D.C. in Tulsa

> Dear D.C.: It's neither. It's whom you know.

One should know for *whom* the bell tolls. It tolls for thee. The first time I see the title of Hemingway's book as "For Who the Bell Tolls," or a letter starting "To Who It May Concern," I'll throw in the towel.

In the meantime, despite the lazy writer's insistence on using *who* in every context, I'll continue to teach that *whom* should be used when it is the object of a preposition or a sentence and in other places where the objective (accusative) case is called for. However, this rule presupposes a flair or an ear for the language. For this reason alone, correct usage of *who* and *whom* may already be an L.C.

Parenthetical phrases—or those that could be set off by commas—should not influence the case of a pronoun, in these instances *who* and *whoever*:

> Write to the one who you know is the senior author of the article.
>
> The government will investigate whoever they believe was responsible for the ecologic catastrophe.
>
> These physicians studied a 45-year-old man who they were sure had Alzheimer's disease.

Keep your concentration fixed on the subject of the verb. In the first example, without the parenthetical material it would correctly read "who is the senior author"; in the second, "whoever was responsible."

In many instances there is a practical way to know whether to use *who* or *whom*: Try replacing the *who* or *whom* with *he* or *him*. If *he* is wrong, so is *who*. The same for *him*; if it's wrong, so is *whom*.

> Who do you consider the best hematologist?

Try turning the sentence around: "Do you consider *him* the best hematologist?" Since *him* is correct and *he* would be incorrect, *whom* is the proper choice.

The *New York Times Winners & Sinners* suggests an easy mnemonic device: The words that end in *m* are interchangeable. If it should be *him* or *them*, it should be *whom*.

CHAPTER 6

Loose Use

ADMINISTER

Probably because *administrate* sounds more stately, some people use it rather than *administer*. The two words are synonymous but not interchangeable. The shorter and plainer word is always preferable.

Both words are from the same Latin root, *administrare* (*ad* + *ministrare*, "to attend" or "manage." *Ministrare* means "to serve."

It is idiomatic to write "administer [not administrate] first aid."

Webster III quite simply gives *administer* as the synonym for *administrate* and cites many examples of usage for *administer* but none for *administrate*.

> The physician determines the amount of antivenin to be administered [not administrated].

Unfortunately, the intransitive verb *minister* (to) in the sense of "serve" is obsolescent except in certain professions or occupations. *Minister* is seen only in a context of compassion; thus my use of *unfortunately*. There is little enough compassion in the world as it is.

> Their mission was to minister to the sick and the poor in their own cities.

Administer is a transitive verb and therefore can take an object.

> Cardiac nurses administer medications to patients with heart disease at carefully planned and monitored intervals.

The noun *administration* (usually followed by *of*) has many meanings; it can refer to, *inter alia*, justice, blows, regimes or terms of office, discipline, medicine, funds, public affairs, management, the performance of executive duties, oaths, sacraments, estates, trusts, governments, and persons responsible for managing a business, institution, or other endeavor.

AGGRAVATE

Arthritis, particularly of the knee, is sometimes aggravated by obesity.

To *aggravate* is to make worse. People cannot be aggravated. Conditions or situations can be. People can be provoked, irritated, irked, incensed, annoyed, or exasperated.

AUTHORED

This word is often used as an alternative to *wrote*, but it is substandard. Real writers, who seldom refer to themselves as authors, just write—they don't author.

Nevertheless, the writers of plays should proudly step onto the stage when the audience shouts "Author! Author!"

CENTER AROUND

It is impossible for anything to *center around* anything else; the center is the center, and everything else is around it:

All of their research was centered on the activity of the spirochete.

COMPENDIUM

Although *compendium* has a capacious ring to many, it actually means a brief compilation, an outline or abridgment, not a comprehensive work:

To save valuable time, pharmacists use compendiums of proprietary and nonproprietary drugs every day.

When they need more details than they can garner from a short work such as a compendium, they often refer to a monograph on a particular preparation or to a book on pharmacology.

FEWER, LESS

In general, *fewer* has to do with number and *less* with mass or quantity:

The blood specimen contained fewer leukocytes than normal.
There may be less glory in some professions than others, but their practitioners find great satisfaction in them nonetheless.

Using *fewer* in the right context is not an affectation; it's just good usage.

FRACTIONS AND PARTS THEREOF

A mistake of 0.6 centimeters can skew the experiment.

Since 0.6 would be spelled out six-tenths of *a* or *one centimeter*, the singular should have been used in that sentence: "0.6 *centimeter*."

Tolerances of less than .24 *inch* are common in diemaking.

INCOMPARABLES

The United States Constitution speaks of a "more perfect union." As an incomparable, *perfect* cannot be modified or qualified, although one may correctly use "almost perfect" or "nearly perfect." Maybe people in the Revolutionary War era didn't regard *perfect* as an incomparable.

In *Julius Caesar*, Shakespeare referred to the stabbing of Caesar as the "most unkindest cut of all." However, he too may be excused for a seemingly ungrammatical glitch. As was the custom then, he and his contemporaries often used the older form, *most*, along with the newer *-est* suffix. In time, the suffix became the vogue and was used more and more often by itself.

In our day, we use either *most* or *-est,* since both are correct as the superlatives of adjectives. Cadence and rhythm usually govern the choice. This presupposes a good ear for language. *Commonest,* for example, is correct, but I generally use *most common,* because it falls more pleasantly on my ear—a purely subjective judgment.

These forms are called *double comparatives* ("more perfect") or *double superlatives* ("most unkindest"). They would more correctly be termed *uncomparables,* since they cannot be compared. *Incomparable* denotes things that are without equal. However, the distinction is often overlooked, and most writers have never used *uncomparable.*

Other incomparable adjectives (absolutes) include *absolute, best, equal, eternal, fatal, final, least, lethal, supreme, terminal, total, unanimous,* and *worst.*

MINIMIZE, MINIMUM

Some parts of speech other than adjectives are incomparables or absolutes: *minimize* and *maximize* are two absolute verbs. To minimize anything is to take it down to the bare bones, the *least possible* quantity or degree. *Minimize* (from *minimum*) is often misused; verbs such as *decrease, lessen, lower, diminish,* or *reduce* should be used instead.

By the same token, the noun *minimum* (from the Latin *minimus,* least, which is the superlative of *minor,* minor) should be used to express the lowest quantity or the least possible quantity, extent, or degree, not some vague *lower* degree or quantity.

Maximum as a noun means the greatest or highest quantity, extent, or degree. It can also be used as an adjective with the same sense, although I prefer to use the better adjective *maximal.*

RELATIONS, RELATIONSHIPS

> The subject admitted to having a homosexual relationship with "Joe" in the eighth-floor hotel corridor.

What these men were having was homosexual relations. A one-night stand does not a relationship make.

> What is often overlooked in long-term hospitalization is the importance of the nurse-patient relationship.

A relationship denotes interconnectedness; it is the state of being related or interrelated. *Relation* in most of its meanings is already an abstract, although it does have a concrete meaning in the sense of "narration." The suffix *-ship* is from an Old High German word, and ultimately a prehistoric Germanic word, meaning condition, nature, or quality; it makes concretes of abstracts: *sibship, kinship.*

This suffix also denotes dignity, profession, or skill, as in *authorship, clerkship, deanship,* and *scholarship,* or a quality or state of being, as in *courtship* and *fellowship.*

TANDEM

> In this sentence, *tandem* is used incorrectly:

> Psychotherapists there work in tandem with occupational and recreational therapists.

Tandem is directly from the Latin, meaning literally "at length," taken to mean "lengthwise." It does not mean side by side, abreast, or yoked together. Consider the tandem bicycle: The riders, two or more, are one behind the other. *Indian file* is a synonym for *tandem.*

> The 100 hikers are climbing Mt. Rainier in tandem.

There is no limit to the number of people, animals, or things that can be in tandem.

In London I saw at least 30 people patiently waiting in tandem for a bus.

VICIOUS CIRCLE

The phrase, by now an oft-misused cliche, is *vicious circle,* not *vicious cycle.*

The first patient was a young man trapped in the vicious circle of anxiety-fatigue-anxiety.

One may well inquire why a cycle can't be as vicious as a circle. Maybe it can. However, I refuse to think of the Krebs cycle as vicious; my mind blocks right there. I've never seen an instance in which *vicious cycle* would be correct; invariably it should have been *vicious circle.*
Cornelia Evans and Bergen Evans wrote:

Vicious in this context [logic] means impaired or spoiled by a fault. *Circle* means a mode of reasoning wherein a proposition is used to establish a conclusion and then this same conclusion used to prove the proposition. It is called a circle because it has no real starting place—and, one might add, because there's no end to this sort of thing. It is one of the most popular of all fallacies, the darling of the pompously ignorant. The term *vicious circle* is commonly used to describe a situation in which solution of one problem creates other problems whose solution is incompatible with the original circumstances.

The entry in *Webster III* under *vicious circle principle* is as follows:

A principle in logic: whatever is defined in terms of all of a collection or of a totality cannot be a member thereof—compare [Bertrand] Russell's paradox.

Although *circle* and *cycle* are ultimately from much the same roots, they have unrelated meanings and usages. Nevertheless, that is not to say that someone, somewhere, somehow won't come up with a correct example of a *vicious cycle* (a wobbly penny-farthing?).

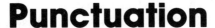

CHAPTER 7

Punctuation

In this chapter I discuss a few kinds of punctuation. For intricate detail on the subject, I suggest consulting an up-to-date book on grammar.

APOSTROPHES

ELISION

One use of the apostrophe is to indicate an omission of letters (elision) in a word.

> You're (you are) late for your appointment at the clinic.
> She's (She has) been waiting for her deanship for some time.

Theoretically that could mean either "she is" or, slangily or colloquially, "she has." Since "she is been waiting" is not good English, the inference must be that "she has been waiting" is meant.

Sometimes the apostrophe and *s* are used incorrectly:

> It's pharmacologic properties make it suitable for geriatric patients as well.

"It is pharmacologic properties" is certainly wrong. "It's" *never* means anything but "it is" or (colloquially) "it has." This error is seen often in (mis)translation into English; there is no reason for native English writers to make it.

> If you're siblings are equally at risk, it would be better to have them vaccinated as well.

"You're" *never* means anything but "you are." Write "*your* siblings."

> ... who's broad stripes and bright stars, through the perilous fight ...

"Who's" is short for "who is." "*Whose* broad stripes and bright stars" is correct.

The misuse of the apostrophe immediately stamps the writer as uncultured and just this side of illiterate—not a reputation she or he wants.

POSSESSIVES OF NOUNS

The possessive case of a singular noun, whether ordinary or proper, is formed by adding an apostrophe and *s*, no matter what the last consonant or sound in the word happens to be.

> The technician proceeded with the testing despite the batch's appearance.
>
> Elizabeth's eyes are brown; the lenses are violet.
>
> Because of the trauma, the internist was concerned about James's spleen.

Sibilants are *s*, *sh*, *ch*, or *z* sounds. The fact that *lens* and other nouns or proper nouns end in a sibilant does not change the rule.

> The lens's other names are "crystalline humor" and "crystalline lens."

There are exceptions. Because of tradition and for euphony, some singular nouns add only the apostrophe for the possessive:

> for goodness' sake
> for righteousness' sake
> for conscience' sake

The names *Moses* and *Jesus* are made possessive by adding an apostrophe but not an *s*:

> out of Moses' land
> in Jesus' name

When names end in silent *s*, *x*, or *z*, the possessive is made by adding an apostrophe and *s*, in the usual way:

> Dumas's characters
> Descartes's aphorism
> Agassiz's explorations

Some polysyllabic names, many of them Greek or hellenized, ending in a sibilant or an *-eeze* sound take only an apostrophe for reasons of euphony:

> Eusebius' martyrdom
> Ladislas' regime
> Artaxerxes' campaign
> Archimedes' "eureka"
> Euripides' plays

Hippocrates' teachings

The possessive case of plural nouns is usually made by adding only an apostrophe:

> The lenses' shapes are reproducible.
>
> In time, watchmakers' hands become susceptible to carpal tunnel syndrome.
>
> Dancers' calf muscles tend to become bunchy.

Some irregular plurals take an apostrophe and *s*:

> Men's bones are generally larger than women's.
>
> Infants with special heart, orthopedic, or other problems are transferred to Children's Hospital.

Possessives of closely linked nouns and proper nouns are made by adding an apostrophe and *s* to only the final element:

> Zollinger and Ellison's contributions to gastroenterology
>
> Banting and Macleod's Nobel Prize
>
> Funk and Wagnalls' dictionary
>
> the mother and father's parental obligations

Use of the apostrophe and *s* to make the possessive of proper names of more than one syllable ending in a sibilant is controversial. The preceding examples are generally accepted, but I will understand if some of them are disputed.

POSSESSIVE "OF" UNDERSTOOD

The apostrophe can imply the addition of the word *of* to a phrase:

> What the agency needs is a person with five years' experience in human resources.

The apostrophe in this instance indicates that a person with five years *of* experience is needed.

Sometimes an apostrophe is used when it is not correct:

> At least half of the patients were four months' pregnant.

"Four months of pregnant" is patently incorrect. The apostrophe should be deleted.

The test is to mentally insert *of* between the two words; if *of* is incorrect, so is the apostrophe.

COMMAS

The presence or absence of a comma can change meaning:

Let me call you sweetheart.
Let me call you, sweetheart.

Here is lexicographer Maxwell Nurnberg's famous contribution:

What's the latest dope?
What's the latest, dope?

A comma mistakenly used can cause disasters. Take the "Case of the $2 Million Comma," as cited by Theodore M. Bernstein in his syndicated newspaper column on usage many years ago. Bernstein, who died in 1979, was a professor at the Columbia University School of Journalism and the Assistant Managing Editor (later Consulting Editor) of the *New York Times.*

The "Supreme Court of American Journalism" (a justly deserved honorific accorded Bernstein by Abigail Van Buren and concurred in by many others, mainly editors and writers), told this true story (my paraphrase):

In 1873 the Congress enacted a tariff bill intending to exempt certain products from payment of duty, including "all foreign fruit-plants," that is, *plants* imported for purposes of experimentation, propagation, or transplantation. The clerk who copied the bill mistakenly used a comma [fruit, plants] instead of a hyphen. Until a new version of the act could be printed, *all* foreign fruit and plants were lawfully admitted to U.S. ports duty-free.

The negligence of the clerk (who certainly was no proofreader) cost the United States more than $2 million in revenues.

A missing comma could cause considerable grief:

The suit was filed on behalf of David Hopper, whose leg was broken by his parents, Mr. and Mrs. William Hopper.

If the parents had seen that item in the newspaper, they might have contemplated a libel suit.

APPOSITION

Commas set off appositional (modifying) words or phrases. Here is an incorrect use:

Neurotoxicity is the main limiting side effect of the antitumor agent, vincristine.

The comma in that sentence and the word *the* indicate that there is only one antitumor agent. We all know that there are many such agents, so no comma is needed there. Delete it.

> She was informed that her husband Carl was on duty that day at the base's infirmary.

The lack of a comma there would indicate that she had more than one husband, a potentially bigamous and therefore libelous possibility.

> Tell us whether his brother, Brandon, could be implicated in this scheme to defraud Medicare.

The appositional commas mean that he had only one brother. If there had been no commas, the implication would have been that he had more than one brother.

COMMAS BETWEEN ADJECTIVES

Often the question arises whether the writer should use commas between adjectives:

> Their two efficient young secretaries were given commensurate raises.

There are three adjectives modifying "secretaries." Should there be commas between adjectives? The solution lies in knowing whether the adjectives are coordinate or equal, that is, whether you could insert "and" between them. Could you say "two and young and efficient secretaries" and still have a decent sentence? No; the adjectives are not coordinate, so commas should not be used.

> Lisa was praised as a kind good-hearted pleasant hospital volunteer.

Could you say "kind *and* good-hearted *and* pleasant"? Yes; all the adjectives are coordinate, so there should be commas between them: "kind, good-hearted, pleasant hospital volunteer."

DATES AND COMMAS

The comma is optional but is usually omitted when only a month and a year are given:

> November 1968
> July 14, 1789

SENIOR, JUNIOR, AND THE THIRD

Senior (*Sr.*) and *Junior* (*Jr.*) after a person's name are usually preceded by a comma.

> William Strunk, Jr.
> Wilhelm His, Sr.

However, many house styles omit the preceding comma or the ending period in the abbreviated form.

Other collateral designations such as *2nd, 3rd, the Third, III,* and *IV* are not preceded by a comma.

> Louis XIV
> Pope Pius X
> Charles the Second
> Benjamin Smart 3rd

No, I don't know why. I conjecture that the comma is omitted in these expressions because the numeral is considered an integral part of the name, whereas *Jr.* and *Sr.*, being subject to change upon the demise of Senior, are not. One tenuous analogy might be "John Cardinal O'Hara"; Cardinal is not his middle name.

In passing, I must note that this section does not apply to the designation *Malcolm X.* Malcolm Little was not Malcolm the Tenth; he took this *nom de guerre* as a political and religious tactic and commentary.

SERIAL COMMA

The serial comma—a comma after the penultimate item in an enumeration—is optional. Follow the house style of the publication you're writing for.

Although there is much to be said for the serial comma, its use sometimes causes some head-scratching:

> The two suspects have been charged with robbery, aggravated and simple assault, recklessly endangering others, a weapons offense, and conspiracy.

Does that mean that "recklessly endangering others" is a weapons offense (in apposition) (four charges) or does it mean that "weapons offense" is still another charge (five charges in all)? If the latter, this phrase could have been enclosed in parentheses to avoid ambiguity. Another device is to use semicolons to set off each item, with necessary commas within the item.

> Please state name, age, sex and housing requirements.

That sentence is a good argument for the serial comma.

ELLIPSES

An ellipsis, marked by dots or asterisks, indicates an omission in a sentence or other part of a work.

If the omitted text is within a sentence, the ellipsis (omission) is indicated by three spaced dots (also known as leaders or periods). Always leave a space between the dots and before and after the dots:

> The commissioner was quoted as follows: "Our understanding was that the company had submitted the proper documentation . . . and that all the data were forthcoming."

If the omitted text follows a completed sentence, there should be four dots—the dot (period) indicating the end of the sentence and then the usual three:

> The work of the task force was completed on time. . . . The force has been requested to hand in its report within six months.

In contradistinction to the three-dot ellipsis, there is no space between the last word in the sentence and the first period, the period ending the sentence.

HYPHENS

There is as much variation in opinion among lexicographers and grammarians as among expert witnesses. Furthermore, punctuation "rules" change. Dictionaries—the infrequently published unabridged ones and the more up-to-date ones—may differ as to whether a particular term should be hyphenated or written solid.

The general rule is that when a compound term consisting of two or more words becomes common enough to find its way into written material for a few years, it is first hyphenated and then, after a respectable interval, it becomes solid.

Some terms have become so frequent that even the most conservative practitioner (and I am not one of those) sees fit to bow. Alexander Pope wrote:

> In words, as fashions, the same rule will hold,
> Alike fantastic if too new or old:
> Be not the first by whom the new are tried,
> Nor yet the last to lay the old aside.

Health care is such a term. This phrase is written by most good writers as two words. When it becomes a compound adjective, the question arises as to whether it should be hyphenated. I vote for not hyphenating, because *health care institutions* is unambiguous. *Health-care institutions* is also unambiguous, but the hyphen is unnecessary.

I vote strongly against *healthcare* and other such formulations because I am against teutonization of the language, that is, agglomeration. If we sanction healthcare, a term that reflects the writer's (or the client's) bias, what is to stop anyone from coining "geriatricare," "healthcarepractitioners," "pediatricare," "footcare," or "earcare"? *Und so weiter.*

In the past several years manufacturers and advertisers have considered it clever and chic to join two unrelated words to coin the names of cosmetics, drugs, medical products, computer software, and other branded commodities, and to plunk a capital letter into the middle of the name, with or without a hyphen. Many readers find this practice wearisome and wish the coiners would call a halt to it.

ADVERBS MODIFYING ADJECTIVES

Hyphens are not used in compound adjectival modifiers after adverbs ending in -*ly*. If an adverb not ending in -*ly* could not be misinterpreted as an adjective modifying the noun, don't use a hyphen.

> the highly trained technician
> an individually devised regimen
> the less common cancers
> the most effective medications
> a justly celebrated scientist

Some other compounds made up of adverbs modifying adjectives are hyphenated if they precede the verb. When the compound comes after the verb, the phrase is not hyphenated:

> the ill-advised patient; *but* the patient was ill advised
> a well-defined regimen, *but* the regimen was well defined.

A caveat: Some adjectives end in -*ly*; they should be differentiated from adverbs, and they *do* take a hyphen when they modify other adjectives:

> a disorderly-looking clinic
> the scholarly-appearing report
> pearly-white teeth

CHEMICAL SUBSTANCES AS MODIFIERS

Names of chemical substances used as adjectival modifiers are not usually hyphenated.

> The internist prescribed salicylic acid medication.

A representative of the coroner's office said that the victims had died of carbon monoxide poisoning.

Hyphens are not necessary when the adjectival term is unambiguous.

CLARIFIERS

"When *I* use a word," Humpty Dumpty said, in rather a scornful tone, "it means just what I choose it to mean—neither more nor less."
"The question is," said Alice, "whether you *can* make words mean so many different things."
"The question is," said Humpty Dumpty, "which is to be master—that's all."
—Lewis Carroll, *Through the Looking Glass.*

In writing, as in editing, one important goal is to ease the reader's task in comprehending, and, above all, to avoid ambiguity. Hyphens are used to clarify.

Signing is essential for hearing impaired [hearing-impaired] youngsters.

This stereoscopic angiography system can take three dimensional [three-dimensional] images of blood vessels in the brain.

The hyphens render the sentences immediately intelligible.

The study cohort consisted of 12 year old children.

Did the writer mean a dozen children, each of whom is a year old, or an indeterminate number of children, each of whom is 12 years old? The writer must be queried.

The Massachusetts laboratories had sent 4 day old Sprague-Dawley rats. [Either 4 day-old or 4-day-old; the writer must be queried.]

Poor writing is costly. One can only estimate its cost to American commerce, but one expert puts it at about $1 billion a year. Consider the case of the clerk who damaged expensive radioactive rods beyond repair because of a mangled shipping order. He had the rods cut into 10 one-foot lengths. The order had called for "10-foot-long pieces."

COMPOUND VERBS

Verb forms that end in prepositions or adverbs (compound verbs) should not be hyphenated:

The ambulance took her to the emergency department when she started to black out.

The nurse was forced to turn over her care to the next shift.

Because of a change in administration, they split up the department into four sections.

However, when the same two words are used as nouns, they are written solid or hyphenated:

Her blackout was found to be due to a low blood glucose level.

The maintenance turnover is excessive this year.

After the split-up, conditions improved considerably.

Note that although *out* in the following sentence is the last word, even the people who think it's incorrect to end a sentence with a preposition would be satisfied—*out* in this instance is part of the verb and is not considered a preposition. In such a context, it is usually called an adverb, part of a fused verb form.

All the terms of the contract were spelled out.

Adjectival forms of compound verbs are not hyphenated when they follow a verb, but are hyphenated when they precede their associated nouns:

Everyone in the operating room was worn out by the end of the three-vessel operation.

The worn-out mores of our society must be replaced by more civilized ones.

Each regulation was spelled out in detail.

Spelled-out numbers are often cumbersome in ordinary usage.

FOREIGN PHRASES

Webster III and other dictionaries, as well as books on usage, are excellent guides to the use of hyphens in specific adjectival phrases.

In English, as in other living languages, there is a perpetual drive toward simplification. Some integrated Latin adjectival terms, at one time hyphenated, are now joined: postmortem findings, antenatal examination, postpartum infection (*but* infection post partum). However, certain other Latin phrases are still written as two words, even when they are used as modifiers:

bona fide credentials

de facto head of the department

per diem symposium expenses

pro rata allocation

viva voce vote

IN VITRO, IN VIVO

These Latin terms have been part of the English language, particularly in medical usage, for so long that they have been graduated to nonhyphenation. Medical journals in the nineteenth century did hyphenate them when they were used as modifiers of nouns.

Whether they are used as adjectives or adverbs, in vivo and in vitro are never hyphenated. They are entirely unambiguous without the hyphen in any context.

> These pharmaceuticals were tested extensively in vitro.
>
> Because of the in vivo findings, the FDA approved the investigational drugs in good time.

In vitro and in vivo are not italicized in American English usage, although they used to be. Their italicization in current American medical journals is a sign that the person in charge is not au courant or is intransigent.

MEDICAL CONDITIONS AND ENTITIES

Medical conditions and entities used as modifiers (adjectives) are not usually hyphenated:

> sickle cell trait
>
> squamous cell carcinoma

However, such phrases as *giant-cell tumor* and *soft-tissue area* should be hyphenated, since they would otherwise be ambiguous.

NON-, CO-, -LESS, AND OTHER AFFIXES

Some common prefixes and suffixes (collectively called affixes) are joined without hyphens to the word root:

antibacterial	likewise
armless	midchest
bilateral	nonnegotiable
coauthor	nonsense
coexistence	overwrought
cooperation	postoperative
counterproductive	postprandial
extraterrestrial	posttraumatic
hypersensitivity	predetermined
hypotension	preoperative
interseptal	preterm
intracranial	rebound

semihydrated	twofold (*but* "42-fold")
supernatant	underdeveloped
supramaxillary	ultrasound

Some editors and publishing houses prefer to use a hyphen when two or more of the same vowel adjoin: *anti-infective, intra-aortic.* Nonetheless, their house styles usually call for *reenter* to be written solid. I write them solid.

At one time a dieresis was worn by the *o* in *co-* words, but that's ancient history. The dieresis (*umlaut* in German) indicated that the first two letters of these words were sounded separately from the next letter: koh-operation, not kooperation.

NOUNS COMBINED WITH ADJECTIVES

Cholesterol-induced, accident-prone, and other such phrases are always hyphenated.

Note that in each instance the first element is a noun and not an adjective. A correct term would be *water-soluble,* not *watery-soluble.* Similarly, *endothelium-mediated* is correct, rather than *endothelial-mediated.*

NOUNS LINKED TO NOUNS

Hyphenation between nouns usually indicates that they are of equal value or that they have common characteristics:

> His credentials as a writer-editor were unassailable.
> Lewis Thomas is a physician-author-philosopher par excellence.

Note that the slash mark (virgule, separatrix, solidus) should *not* be used, since it would mean a separation, not a joining. The virgule is overused, misused, and abused. In too many instances it clouds the meaning:

> The endocrinologist stated that the clinical/diagnostic presentation was complicated.

That's not all that's complicated. I can only surmise what the writer meant in that sentence. However, editors and readers should not have to surmise or speculate. It is difficult, if not impossible, to get into someone else's mind (the writer's, in this instance).

PREFIXES AND PROPER NOUNS

A hyphen is used when a proper noun or adjective follows a prefix:

> anti-Semitic quotas

non-European physicians
pre-Leeuwenhoek microscopes
post-Vesalian teachings
pre-Kantian concepts
pro-Semmelweiss group

When -*like* is at the end of an adjective, the word is ordinarily not hyphenated unless the main element ends in two *l*'s or is a proper noun or a proper adjective:

Cochlear means shell-like.
Some hospitals' offices are more businesslike than some businesses' offices.
a Holter-like monitor

RE- WORDS

Some words starting with *re-* should sometimes be hyphenated to obviate ambiguity:

re-creation

To create something once again might be *recreation*, but it is certainly *re-creation*.

re-mark

If changes are made after the first go-around, the proofreader is expected to *re-mark* the galley or page proofs.

re-solve

In that television series, the medical examiner was often able to *re-solve* a homicide mystery.

SPELLED-OUT WORDS AND NUMERALS

The hyphen is not used in spelled-out words, but is used with numerals:

tenfold
3.5-fold
14-fold

UNHEALTHFUL HYPHENS

Hyphens that are omitted can be lethal, or, at the least, can have deleterious effects:

> The oncologist had prescribed 6 mercaptopurine tablets 50 mg b.i.d.

What the oncologist had actually prescribed was one 50 mg 6-mercaptopurine tablet twice a day. Let us hope that this error was detected in time.

Note that hyphens are not used in a term such as *50 mg,* even though it is a compound adjective modifying *tablet.*

Lethal hyphens are companions to "Decimals That Kill" (in Chapter 4, "Medical and Pharmaceutical Pointers").

The last thing the professions need is more malpractice suits.

THE WORD PROCESSOR AND HYPHENATION

As explained in Chapter 4 (section on "Justified Lines in Manuscripts"), in medical work it is advisable to instruct the word processor operator never to hyphenate at the end of a line of text or at the end of a page. It is far better not to justify lines of text (nonjustification in this context is called "ragged right margin").

If lines have been justified in a manuscript, the editor should draw a ligature and a slash through the hyphen to indicate to the typesetter that the hyphen at the end of the line merely indicates syllabication (if, indeed, this is the case). Otherwise, the word could be mistakenly printed as a compound, hyphenated word. Most journals frown on justified lines in manuscripts, mainly because justification makes it difficult to calculate the number of words in a manuscript.

What is the typesetter to make of the following sentence?

> Whatever the problem is with the new
> wing, the solution is not under-
> development.

Maybe the solution is overdevelopment. Only the writer knows for certain.

When a hyphen at the end of a line is to be retained, as in *self-explanatory* and other such terms, the editor should so indicate by adding a line under the hyphen to make an equals sign (=, the editorial notation for hyphen) of it.

YEAR-LONG

Terms such as *year-long* and *month-long* should be hyphenated, not written solid. That time may come, but it's not here yet—at least not for me.

PARENTHESES

If a parenthetic phrase refers to and is part of the sentence, the period of the sentence should come after the parentheses:

There was no effect on the heart rate (Fig. 1).
Body weight remained the same throughout the study (see Table 1).

If the entire sentence is enclosed within parentheses, the period is always inside the ending parenthesis:

The electrolyte imbalance was observed soon after the medication was administered. (See the bar graph for details.)

Occasionally an incorrect hybrid is seen:

There was no effect on the heart rate. (Fig. 4)

The allusion to the figure should be within the relevant antecedent sentence:

There was no effect on the heart rate (Fig. 4).

I landmark figures and tables in the margin at first mention. It is also my editorial practice to use *see* "(see Fig. 4)" only if Figure 4 has been previously mentioned in the text. This saves my time and obviates confusion on the part of the journal's production people as to where Figure 4 is first mentioned and therefore located in the text.

PERIODS

As with all other kinds of punctuation, the uses of periods are so numerous that entire chapters of textbooks are devoted to them.

Questioners often want to know whether it's "correct" to omit periods in certain terms, remarking that these terms look strange to them:

S aureus
PhD
MD

They look strange to me too. Having been taught that these abbreviations take periods, and having used periods all of my professional life, I find it disconcerting to see them without periods. In 30 years or so (I should live so long), this practice may not seem bizarre at all. The American Medical Association's house style calls for omission of the period in all its publications; some other organizations follow the same practice.

Stedman's and *Dorland's* include the period in *S. aureus*, M.D., and other such abbreviations. *Webster III* also uses the period—for example, in the abbreviation for *Escherichia coli*, *E. coli.*

I cannot bring myself to omit the familiar period, not so much because it *is* familiar but because without it mistakes will be made that ought not to be made. It's inevitable. Handwriting in particular could be confusing. Os (mouth) could be misread for O.S. (oculus sinister, left eye).

My personal style is to retain the period. Let the microchips fall where they may.

See also the section on "Points and Periods" in Chapter 4, "Medical and Pharmaceutical Pointers."

QUOTATION MARKS

The rules about punctuation and quotation marks are simple.

The American style is to place quotation marks outside the punctuation, even if the quotation contains only one word at the end of a sentence. There are two exceptions, colons and semicolons—unless the colon or the semicolon is in the original quotation.

> Poliomyelitis is almost always shortened to "polio."
>
> The certificate stated that the patient's death was due to a "cerebral vascular accident"; however, the medical examiner was authorized to perform an autopsy.
>
> A hospital spokesperson said that the "next press conference will provide more detail concerning the president's condition": when the operation was performed and how extensive it may be.

Question marks can be either inside or outside the quotation, according to the sense:

> As to the transplant, how long do you think the family will take to "think it over"?
>
> The question is, "What are the risk factors?"

The British style of quotation is different from the American. When in Great Britain, do as the British do. In the United States, follow the seemingly illogical but traditional style of punctuation with quotations. It has served well.

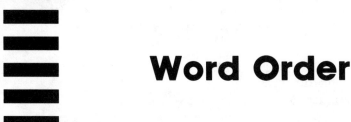

CHAPTER 8

Word Order

Is word order really important? These examples make the point that correct word order is tremendously important for clarity and instant intelligibility. In addition, it decreases the possibility of committing absurdities:

> Hastings has been treated there since the shooting by plastic surgeons and psychologists.
>
> Films taken in the erect or lateral decubitus position will reveal free air in the peritoneal cavity.
>
> The university's president has been asked to resign because of sexual harassment and mismanagement.
>
> Other winners in the awards for journalistic achievement included a report on the slaying of a masseuse by John Shandy of the *Jamestown Herald*.
>
> The optometrist's brochure was full of information on intraocular lenses for nurses.
>
> A 15-year-old girl won the right to play hockey with boys in Quebec Superior Court Wednesday.

Is it any wonder that Canadians are so expert at the game?

> The syndrome, originally attributed to tuberculosis, occurs most commonly in young persons with no sexual predilection.
>
> An appendectomy was performed under general anesthesia.
>
> The patient was first seen two years ago by the primary care physician in a severely debilitated condition.

Which one was in the debilitated condition, the patient or the physician? The reader should not have to guess or reread the sentence.

> The new floor sections will enable babies to be born in Grace Hospital for the first time.
>
> Although other sisters have attended West Point in the past, this is the first time they have been Jewish.
>
> Newspaper advertisement: Free refreshments prepared while you wait in microwave ovens.

Theodore Bernstein's comment about the free refreshments: "Customers who would be willing to wait in those ovens would not be well-done or medium; they would be rare. . . . Every piece of writing should be read a second time to be sure it says what you meant it to say."

> The third-baseman admitted to an affair while standing next to the Cleveland Stadium batting cage.
> Headline: Baby bitten 150 times by rats in good condition.
> The Unknown Warrior in Westminster was brought from Flanders in 1920 and interred in earth brought from the battlefields under the floor of the nave of Westminster.
> What is needed is a list of specialists broken down by specialization.
> In the midst of the confusion, Martin Stone was born next door to Janet Stone, his 19-year-old mother.

That must have taken some fancy footwork.

> Princess Grace announced to Cassini her plans to marry Prince Rainier aboard the Staten Island Ferry.

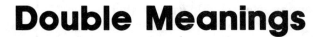

CHAPTER 9

Double Meanings

Many medical writers, notably physicians, assume that the rules of "creative" writing do not apply to their work. Medical writing, they maintain, is expository and formal, and therefore should be pedestrian so as to establish credibility.

All writing is by definition creative, even if it is also expository. The writer has power to impart a group of ideas. It is the writer's obligation to impart it clearly, without ambiguity and, preferably, with elegance and style.

In this chapter I discuss some hazards of ambiguity. Other examples are scattered throughout the book.

The good writer will write so clearly that the reader will never have to read a sentence twice to discover its true meaning. Poets have the right to demand that kind of attention from readers—medical writers do not.

In this book I take it for granted that writers and editors are intellectually honest and that any ambiguity is therefore unintentional or inadvertent.

Writers should adopt the habit of proofreading what they have typed so that double meanings will not hamper the intelligibility of their work.

The laughter usually evoked by the improper use of *in another vein* or other such phrases lasts only a moment. The mischief this kind of error causes may last a great deal longer.

AND/OR

Careful editors will always change the structure of a sentence containing the outmoded phrase *and/or*. Lawyers, who were probably responsible for the use of this term initially, should spell out the possibilities instead of using what some consider a legitimate shortcut.

> The subjects were randomly assigned to receive drug A and/or drug B.

Good medical writers prefer to write instead ". . . or . . . or both." This method adds only a few more characters and obviates ambiguity.

> The subjects were randomly assigned to receive either drug A or drug B, or both.

As Follett points out, everyone knows that if the "weathercaster" says we may have rain or snow tomorrow, it is entirely possible that we may have both. When the chair of the meeting asks whether there are any corrections or additions to the minutes, we know that there may be both.

If it is crucial to exclude one or the other, the writer, whether attorney-at-law or physician, should write "either . . . or . . ."

Follett goes on to say that if those who use *and/or* were as logical as they hope we perceive them to be, they would have to say *and or or*, "since their assumption is that the two cannot coexist."

The above-mentioned phraseology to the contrary notwithstanding, I rise to the defense of lawyers—and their language. The use of "doublets" to reinforce goes way back. In England many centuries ago, when the populace was not as well educated as it is now, it was necessary to use both the common or Anglo-Saxon root word and the French or Latin root word: will and testament; indemnify and hold harmless; lawful and wedded; amounts and denominations; law or statute. Thus the lawyer could use the technical legal term, which would be understood by fellow-lawyers, and the less educated client could understand the plainer term.

Choices have been expressed in English since the fourteenth century without this crutch. *And/or* is a lazy and imprecise way to express alternatives. This borrowing from the special language of law should at last plead *nolo contendere.*

IN ANOTHER VEIN

A Janusian phrase to avoid is *in another vein.* The danger of using it loosely is evident. Hospital technicians in particular should avoid it unless they're serious about it: "Let's try this needle in another vein."

IN ANY CASE

To the average reader, *in any case* may mean "in any event" or "in any circumstances." In medical works, however, *case* refers to the entire history of a patient, living or dead.

> In the worst case, exposure to hydrogen peroxide would be better than continuous exposure to therapeutic solutions containing benzalkonium chloride.

Does that sentence mean "in the worst *of cases*" or "in the worst *event*"? It makes a difference.

Avoid *in any case* in all cases.

Patients should not be referred to as *cases*: "the *patient* in Room 403," not "the *case* [or the appendectomy] in Room 403."

LIKE, SUCH AS

Pharmaceutical writers sometimes write "drugs like diazapam" when they mean "drugs *such as* diazapam." The ambiguity of *like* in this context may create mischief. In the first phrase, the use of *like* may be interpreted as meaning that diazepam is excluded, whereas *such as* specifically includes that drug, as well as other tranquilizers having similar formulas and effects.

OPERATION

Operation usually means a surgical operation, but medical writers should take care to differentiate between that kind and, for example, a computer operation during the surgical operation.

Physicians and nurses generally use spinoffs of *operative* in a surgical context: *preoperative, intraoperative* (meaning "during an operation"), and *postoperative.*

PATENCY, PATENT

Patency and its derivatives should be used cautiously, since they can refer either to "openness" or "clear evidence." If a fistula is *patent*, does that mean that it is open or that the evidence of a fistula is plain?

SIGNIFICANT

Significant is defined as "having meaning." That's all it means. The question the medical writer or editor should ask is, what kind of meaning? Is the finding merely important or is it, for example, statistically significant? In most instances, the author can provide the statistically significant information; the probability (P) value would be helpful too.

Medical writers should be wary of using *significant* unless it is appropriately modified. *Clinically significant* may look profound, but it is so vague—unless amplified—as to be of little value. *Significant* sentences should be restructured to describe the effect:

> As to familial hypercholesterolemia, which calls for a lifetime of therapy, less than optimal compliance to long-term repetitive plasmapheresis may prove a significant factor.

How was the factor significant? Was the effect favorable or adverse? A second look indicates a probability that it was the latter, but the reader should not have to guess.

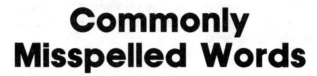

CHAPTER 10

Commonly Misspelled Words

SPELLING IN ENGLISH

The spelling of English is erratic, illogical, and difficult; it is impossible for a foreigner to learn except by constant reading of English-language material or intensive study. Many European languages are phonetic or almost so.

Try explaining to a non-American why *ghoti* (word play attributed to George Bernard Shaw) is pronounced "fish": *gh* as in rough; *o* as in women; and *ti* as in fiction. Or why all these words rhyme, although they're all spelled differently: *complain, champagne, reign, vein, campaign, pane.*

Even geniuses, self-styled and otherwise, may have the disorder known as *malorthographitis,* poor spelling. It is not known whether this is genetically determined, familial, or congenital, but it is endemic in the United States.

The medical profession is uncertain as to whether this disorder can be cured or whether it may some day be prevented by vaccination. In the meantime, the writing, editing, and publishing professions can palliate this dread syndrome. One remedy is in the form of dictionaries written especially for bad spellers—surely an inexpensive prescription for such a costly disorder. The entries in these books are phonetic, so that poor spellers (and I do pity them) can find the words if they can pronounce them. Poor pronouncers will have to undergo an even more difficult course of treatment.

Philosophy and *physician* will undoubtedly be found in that kind of dictionary under *f.*

Which of these words are misspelled?

accomodation	erythematosis
barbituates	foreward
callus	liquify

millenium	stationary
occuring	thru
preceed	vocal chords
pruritis	

Before I discuss this list of words, I have a suggestion for those who are at a loss as to whether one should double a consonant before the final syllable of a word, whether adding a prefix to a word changes the base, and other whethers in spelling English words:

One day, when you're concentrating well, sit down comfortably with the "Spelling" section of *Webster's Third New International Dictionary, Unabridged* (pp. 21a–24a) and read it carefully. Then read the other explanatory notes in the front of the volume (pp. 13a–20a; 25a–54a); it will be most rewarding and professionally enriching.

ACCIDENTALLY

In speech, the penultimate syllable of this word is often clipped, so that it is mispronounced as if it were spelled "accidently." That's probably the reason for the misspelling.

ACCOMMODATION

Like its related word *commode, accommodation* contains two *m*'s. Just remember two *c*'s and two *m*'s.

ACKNOWLEDGMENT

There are only a few words in English that do not ordinarily have an *e* after the *g* in the penultimate syllable, although the *e* is not wrong. *Acknowledgment* is one of them. Some others are *abridgment, fledgling, lodgment*, and *judgment*.

British style usually retains the *e* after the *g*.

AGGRESSIVE

Aggressive management of this disorder may eradicate it early.

Two *g*'s and two *s*'s, please.

ALL RIGHT

This is one of the most commonly misspelled terms in the language.

Despite the descriptive, permissive listing of "alright" as "in reputable use" in at least one unabridged dictionary, I consider it illiterate. *All right* will always be all right with me, and "alright" will always be alwrong.

BARBITURATES

If this word is mispronounced "barbituates," it's no wonder it's also misspelled. The second *r* should also be sounded.

BELLWETHER

> Sloan-Kettering Memorial Hospital became the bellweather in this form of therapy.

A *wether* is a sheep (usually a castrated one) and has little if anything to do with the weather. A *bellwether* is a belled sheep (with a bell around its neck) that is used as leader of the flock.

BIANNUAL, BIENNIAL

Biannual and *semiannual* are virtually synonymous: They both mean twice a year.
Biennial means every other year.

BOOKKEEPER

Not many words in the English language can boast three consecutive twin letters. This is one of them.
All the physician's office manager has to remember is that *bookkeeper* has two *o*'s, two *k*'s, and two *e*'s—but especially two *k*'s.

CALLUS

> The noun *callus* is to be differentiated from *callous*, the adjective.

> The calluses on the champion's hands came from years of playing golf without gloves.

A *callus* is a thickening of the epidermis, usually caused by constant external pressure or friction.

> Sociopaths are characterized by their callous attitude toward other people.

Sociopathic people have a disregard and lack of sympathy for the feelings of others and are indifferent to their sufferings.

CATHETERIZATION

This polysyllabic word is often mistakenly written as "catherization," probably because it is so often mispronounced.

A dye was injected into the patient's arteries in the catheterization laboratory.

CONCERT

Most dermatologists believe that these emollients should be used in consort with the epithelializing ointment.

That should read "in *concert* with," which means "together with." *In consort* sounds as if it should mean "together," and it does, but the phrase carries an implication of mere accompaniment. *In concert* carries the implication of harmony or concord.

Saturday night concerts and Victoria's Prince Consort should help you to keep these two phrases straight.

CORPUS DELICTI

That's what the medical examiner must have to make a determination as to the manner of death.

It is often misspelled or misspoken as "corpus delecti."

The *corpus delicti* can be two things: the body of evidence and the body itself. The plural, should the need arise (may the police force forfend!), is *corpora delicti*.

DEARTH

The commission is studying the dirth of physicians in rural or semirural areas.

The correct spelling is *dearth*. Possibly the writer was unconsciously associating it with girth, which is completely unrelated to the truly troublesome paucity of practitioners, or with mirth, notably absent in such a context.

DE RIGUEUR

This French adjectival phrase refers to a prescribed custom, mode of dress, or etiquette, particularly among people in the more refined strata of society:

An exchange of business cards is *de rigueur* in the Orient, especially among professionals.

EMBARRASS

Bad spelling is an *embarrassment*. This word always has two *r*'s and two *s*'s.

ERLENMEYER FLASK

Because of association with Ehrlich, Ehrenreich, and other such Germanic names, this piece of laboratory equipment is sometimes misspelled "Ehrlenmeyer."

The flask is conical, with a broad, flat bottom; the laboratory worker can shake the flask from side to side without spilling the contents.

Emil Erlenmeyer, the German chemist for whom the flask is named, lived from 1825 to 1909.

ERYTHEMATOSUS

See "Lupus erythematosus."

FOREWORD

There is either *forward* or *foreword*. There is no English word spelled "foreward."

Forward is the antonym of *backward*. The *foreword* to a book, for example, is literally "the word before"; it is usually written by someone other than the author of the book. The preface of a book is written by the author. Some books contain both a foreword and a preface.

FUCHSINOPHILIC

This word is often misspelled "fuschinophilic," probably because of the distorted (inaccurate) pronunciation. Related words, such as *fuchsia*, are frequently misspelled, with the same transposition of letters. Fuchsin acid is also called Acid Violet 19 (*Merck Index*).

> Such easily stained cells are termed fuchsinophilic [having an affinity for the dye].

This famous stain is named after Leonhard Fuchs, a German botanist (1501–1566). Leonard, Leon, or Lionel Fox would be an anglicized equivalent of his name.

HARASS

This word contains only one *r*. It is correctly pronounced with the accent on either the second syllable or, preferably, on the first syllable to obviate sheepishness.

Harass comes from the French *harasser* and Middle French *harer*, "to set a dog on."

HOFFMANN-LA ROCHE AND OTHER OFTEN-MISSPELLED NAMES

The misspelling of the name of this much-respected pharmaceutical house is a constant source of irritation to me and, I'm sure, other editors. The misspelling of a name is unforgivable. I've seen it misspelled in so many different ways, even in otherwise well-edited publications, that when I do see it right, I mentally congratulate the writer or the editor. And yes, there is a space between La and Roche.

Another often misspelled name is *Hoechst-Roussel*. For some reason, hardly anyone misspells the second element; the first part of this hyphenated name is sometimes misspelled "Hoescht," probably because to Americans the combination *sch* is more familiar than *chs*.

Finding the correct spelling of a name, especially the name of a company that figures so prominently in the medical and pharmaceutical fields, is the easiest of editorial tasks.

The *Physicians' Desk Reference* (*PDR*), which includes a partial list of pharmaceutical manufacturers (those who advertise in it), springs to mind as a source first of all. Then there are the *American Drug Index*, the *Merck Index*, and every medical or other library in the world. Try the Mercantile Division of your library if all else fails. For the good editor or writer, there quite simply is no excuse.

Incidentally, even an easy name, *The Upjohn Company*, is sometimes rendered incorrectly. I've seen it spelled "UpJohn." Fancy, but incorrect.

IN MEMORIAM

In memoriam, in invidiam, and *ad nauseam* all end with *-am. In aeternum, in perpetuum, in testimonium,* and *ad infinitum* end in *-um*.

Writers and editors should take 30 seconds to look up the correct spelling of all such phrases. That precaution at the outset may obviate many minutes spent later correcting the galley proof, the page proof, their equivalents, or the "blueline."

INCIDENTALLY

It's no wonder this word is misspelled—it's almost always mispronounced. The penultimate syllable -al should be sounded clearly, even if the a gets the schwa sound.

The *schwa* (no relation to me) is an upside-down *e*, used as a pronunciation mark in dictionaries. It represents a faint, indistinct, unstressed internal vowel sound, like the *e* in *quiet*.

INOCULATE, INNOCUOUS

Many writers misspell *inoculate* with two *n*'s, because they associate it with *innocuous*. Etymologically these two words have nothing in common.

Inoculate—to implant a disease into an organism by introducing the causative agent into it—comes from the Latin (L.) prefix *in-* (meaning in, toward, inward, within) plus L. *oculus*, meaning "eye" or "bud."

Innocuous, meaning "harmless," is formed from the Latin privative prefix *in-* (meaning not) plus *nocuus*, from *nocere*, which you will recognize as part of the famous medical dictum, *Primum non nocere*—First, do no harm.

KREBS CYCLE

This cyclic sequence of reactions, also known as the citric acid or tricarboxylic acid cycle, is sometimes misspelled Kreb's.

The Krebs cycle is named after the English biochemist Sir Hans Adolph Krebs, who earned the 1953 Nobel Prize (with F. A. Lipmann) in Physiology or Medicine for its discovery.

The apostrophe and *s* are not necessary in terms describing tests and cycles. However, if one wishes to use the possessive, it should be *Krebs*' or *Krebs*'s.

LIQUEFY

In the entire English language, there are only four words that end in -*efy*: *liquefy, putrefy, rarefy,* and *stupefy*.

All the other words that have that pronunciation end in -*ify*.

LUPUS ERYTHEMATOSUS

Lupus erythematosis is a devastating disease to those who suffer the facial disfigurement and the systemic effects.

This disorder is systemic lupus erythematos*us*.

Lupus means pike (the fish) or wolf; *erythematosus* refers to inflammatory redness or flushing of the skin. It comes from the Greek *erythema*, flush (skin, not cards), and *erythros*, red.

MALABSORPTION AND ASSIMILATION

This word is often misspelled "malabsorbtion," a form that may seem logical because of the root *absorb*. However, assimilation has taken place here—from *b* to *p*. The Latin word *absorptus* is the past participle of *absorbere*, to absorb.

Assimilation (this kind has to do with etymology, not the gastrointestinal tract) also operates when the privative prefix *in-* changes to *il-*, *im-*, or *ir-* to match the first sound of the next syllable: *illogical, imprecise, irrelevant.*

MILLENNIUM

Their civilization goes back many millenia.

The proper spelling is millen*n*ia, with two *l*'s and two *n*'s. Just think of a*nn*ual.

A *millennium* is a thousand years. "The millennium" is sometimes used to mean the perfect age, free of human imperfections and fostering supreme happiness.

MINUSCULE

Although some dictionaries (not the *OED*, I'm pleased to see) contain the entry "miniscule," many writers consider this variant substandard.

Minuscule is from *minusculus*, which means "somewhat small" and is the diminutive of *minor*. Ultimately *minuscule* is from the Latin comparative *minus*, meaning less, of the adverb *parum*, meaning too little or not enough. *Parum* is from the same root as *parvus*, small; the comparative of *parvus* is *minor* and the superlative *minimus*, meaning least or smallest.

As an adjective, *minuscule* means small or very small. As a noun it is described in the study of paleography as small, cursive writing differing from (the larger) *majuscule*.

Minuscule is also used in printing to denote a lowercase letter.

MUCUS, MUCOUS

The adjective, *mucous*, is often seen when the noun, *mucus*, should have been used.

Mucus contains sloughed-off cells, leukocytes, and inorganic salts.

Mucous membranes are thin sheets of tissue that line and protect the digestive tube, the genitourinary tract, the respiratory passages, and innumerable other anatomic parts.

OCCURRING

The invariable spelling of this word is *occurring*, with two *c*'s and two *r*'s. Ditto for its variants:

Syncope is a frequent occurrence among older patients who have low blood pressure.

OPHTHALMOLOGY

Considering the ubiquity of this word, especially in medical publications, it is surprising to find it so often misspelled, that is, without the first *h*.

Words such as *optic* and *optometry* are always correctly spelled.

Ophthalmology and related terms are from the Greek *ophthalmos*, meaning eye.

Optics and *optometry* are from the Latin *opticus* and the Greek *optikos*, both meaning of or for sight, and the Greek *optos*, seen.

PERQUISITES

This word, abbreviated as "perks" by headline writers and people who don't have the time to pronounce three-syllable words (that's most of us), means privileges or profits, usually associated with employment.

The perquisites of the executive officers included the use of expensive cars, lavish office suites, and junkets abroad.

Perquisite is not to be confused with *prerequisite*, which has a quite different meaning. As one might surmise from the latter word itself, it is something that is required beforehand:

A flair for the language, exactitude, and good judgment are prerequisites for those who aspire to be outstanding editors.

PORTUGUESE

Like *de rigueur*, another oft-misspelled term, this proper name has a *u* after the *g*.

PRECEDE, PROCEED, SUPERSEDE

You need never despair of knowing how to spell these *bêtes noires* and the ramified terms if you can remember four words.

There are only three words in all of English with that sound and in this class that end in *-ceed*: *exceed, proceed,* and *succeed.* There is only one word in English that ends in *-sede*: *supersede.* All others of this class end in *-cede,* including *accede, concede, recede,* and *secede.*

PREDOMINANTLY

The subjects were predominately men over the age of 45.

Predominantly is the proper spelling for this adverb. The verb is *predominate* and the adjective *predominating* or *predominant.*

In human societies, the lawful predominate over the unlawful; this is known as civilization.

The predominating influence is genetic.

PRURITUS

This is one of the most frequently misspelled words in medical works. Inexperienced people assume that all medical words ending with that pronunciation are spelled *-itis. Pruritus* is one of many exceptions. ·

Many patients with diabetes are plagued by pruritus, which is caused by nerve irritation.

Pruri*tus* is pure Latin, from *prurire,* to itch.

RESTAURATEUR

Advertisement by a computer business systems firm: Business owners, physicians, restauranteurs—get a grip on your money, and hang on to it.

This company should have a better grip on spelling. The word is *restaurateur* (no *n*), right out of the French, and Late Latin *restaurator,* meaning restorer, from the Latin *restauratus,* past participle of *restaurare,* to restore.

A *restaurant* is where one goes to restore the inner man or woman by eating wholesome food; a *restaurateur* is the proprietor of such an establishment.

RESUME

The personnel director requested the applicant's resume.

Résumé has *two* acute accents, not one, if you insist on using any. Too often it is misspelled, with only one acute accent, the one over the final *e*. A widely known stationery manufacturer has made this very mistake in its "Resume" series.

The brain makes the leap from verb to noun in accordance with the context, that is, from *resume*—to start again—to *résumé*—a curriculum vitae, or summing up of one's career. Note also that the proper spelling of the synonym is *curriculum vitae, not* "curriculum vita." I have seen this error made on the resumes of Ph.D.'s. The plural is curricula vitae.

A *résumé* is a summary or abstract. It comes from the French *se résumer*, a verb meaning to sum up; a related phrase in French is *en résumé*, meaning in short, or to sum up.

It is no longer necessary to use the acute accents over the two *e*'s, since *resume* is now an integral part of the English language. The same goes for other diacritical marks from all languages if the words or phrases have become a part of the language. It is also not necessary to italicize them.

If there is a moral to this section, it is that you should look up in an authoritative dictionary every unusual word you encounter; don't assume that everything in print is ipso facto correct.

SOLELY

The spelling of this word requires two *l*'s. It is often misspelled "soley," most likely because that's how it sounds.

STATIONARY

This word means standing still, immobile, motionless. The other word, *stationery*, has to do with paper.

The best mnemonic aid I can suggest for *stationary* is right out of pulmonology: st*a*tion*a*ry *a*ir (defined as air that ordinarily stays in the lungs during respiration). The next best one is st*a*tion*a*ry b*a*thtub, right out of my elementary school days.

Stationery is easier: Think of l*e*tt*e*rh*e*ad or *e*nvelop*e*.

STRAITJACKET

The attendants stumbled out of the house, with the patient struggling to escape her straightjacket.

Although the spelling in the preceding sentence is also correct, the more common spelling is *straitjacket.*

THRESHOLD

The oncologist believed that she was on the threshold [not threshhold] of an important advance in the molecular biology of neoplasms.

THROUGH

Despite the best efforts of sign makers and other arbiters of literacy, the word is still spelled *through*, although for how much longer no one can say.

The main advantage of *thru* is its brevity; its main disadvantage is its incorrectness.

VERISIMILITUDE

The occasion may not present itself more than once in a lifetime, but this word should be spelled with all four *i*'s. I once saw a movie review by an eminent critic in which this word was misspelled twice. Once is a typo; twice is poor spelling. By the way, this is the same article in which the critic spelled *de rigueur* "de rigor."

VOCAL CORDS

See the entry "Cord, Chord" in Chapter 12, "Dangerous Dyads and Troublesome Triads."

WITHHOLD

Two *h*'s, please, in this taxing word.

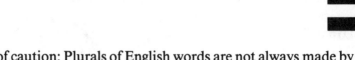

CHAPTER 11

Singular Plurals

A word of caution: Plurals of English words are not always made by adding *s*.

ABBREVIATIONS

Abbreviations for units of measurement are inherently singular or plural: mg, mEq, IU, g, L (for liter) and its ramified forms such as dL and mL, gr (for grain), and innumerable other such terms. Consequently, they remain the same, whether singular or plural.

The plurals of some other abbreviations are discussed in Chapter 18, "Acronyms and Other Abbreviations."

ACOUSTICS AND OTHER -ICS WORDS

What is the plural, if any, of words such as *acoustics, politics,* and *statistics*? These are plural nouns but are either singular or plural in construction—that is, they may take either a singular or a plural verb, depending on the meaning. The rule here is that such *-ics* words take a singular verb if the writer means a subject, as in a college curriculum or a speech, and a plural verb if the writer means to give a practical touch:

> Acoustics is a proper subject for study by architects.
> The acoustics in the surgical amphitheater are excellent.
> Politics makes strange bedfellows.
> The politics in the medical center were too complicated for the new senior resident.
> Statistics was one of the medical student's favorite subjects.
> They went to great lengths to demonstrate that in this study their statistics were valid.

Webster III and other superior unabridged dictionaries will tell you whether such a word is singular or plural and will give you usage notes and examples.

APPENDIX

Since an *appendix* is an appendage, whether to a body or to a book, the plural can be *appendixes* or *appendices*, depending on your preference. One medical dictionary gives both plurals for the anatomic part; another gives only *appendices* as that plural.

CHERUB

The plurals of this heavenly word, which comes directly from Hebrew, are *cherubs* and *cherubim*.

Another celestial word right out of the Hebrew is *seraph*. The plurals are *seraphim* and *seraphs*.

CORPUS LUTEUM

This term, a singular, is a common anatomic term in obstetrics and gynecology. *Corpus* is neuter gender in Latin, and the plural is *not* corpi.

So what could be the plural? Fortunately for those with tight time schedules, one favorite medical dictionary comes to the rescue with the welcome intelligence that the plural is *corpora lutea*. *Lutea*, being a good Latin adjective, agrees with the noun it modifies in number (plural) and gender (neuter).

Progesterone is a hormone secreted by the corpus luteum.

Oh yes. The term literally means yellow body.

CRITERION

Criterion is singular. One cannot adhere to "a criteria." Like other such Greek words that have been integrated into English, the plural is made with an *a* at the end. *Criteria*, being plural, takes a plural verb. *Criterions* is also correct. It just doesn't sound as scholarly.

The principal criterion for physicians is the willingness to work hard.
Antibiotics must meet three U.S.P. criteria: purity, quality, and potency. [I call this the PQP factor.]

DATA, MEDIA

Data and *media* (exactly the same in English as in Latin) are grammatically and etymologically plurals. Consequently, they should take plural verbs. However, this good practice seems to be an L.C.

Many reputable writers and editors now use singular verbs with these words because they reason that although these words are plurals, they could be thought of as constituting a "body of data" or a "group of media." So far I have found it impossible to use singular verbs with these words, and in fact I have never done so.

Datums is used in the fields of topography (for bench marks, as an example) and in mathematics.

Fortunately for my good nature, I have seen *datas* only once or twice, as in "Those [or them] datas are outdated."

Most Latin words that have been thoroughly integrated into English can be pluralized perfectly legitimately by simply adding an *s* to the singular form: *stadiums, memorandums, curriculums.*

Using *stadia, memoranda, curricula, data,* and *media* probably fulfills an honest human need—the need to appear learned.

GENUS

The plural of *genus* (class, group, kind) is *genera.*

The plural of *genius* (an extraordinarily gifted or talented person) is *geniuses* or *genii.*

The plural of *genie* (an imaginary spirit) is *genies* or *genii.*

INSIGNIA

To make life more difficult, the singular in English and Latin is correct as either *insigne* or *insignia*; the plural is either *insignia* or *insignias.*

Every elite corps has its insigne; some have several insignia.

KUDOS

Despite the fact that *kudos* ends in *s*, this Greek word is not a plural—except sometimes. There is no such thing as "a kudo" or "another kudo." There can be more *kudos,* however.

This overused word means accolade, praise, prestige, honor, or renown. *Kudos* can be either singular or plural. However, I've never found out how to use the plural. *Webster III* was no help here—it states that *kudos* is the plural of *kudos*; the examples give no indication of verb number, merely indicating the defined word by that lovely symbol they use, a swung dash.

In addition to kudos, Nobel Laureates receive sums of money, varying with the category and the year.

LOCUM TENENS

A physician or clergyman who substitutes or fills in for someone is a *locum tenens* (plural, *locum tenentes*).

> Although she was originally employed as a locum tenens, the position at the medical center turned out to be permanent.
> Several firms are in the business of placing physicians as locum tenentes.

MICRON

Micron, a unit of length equal to a thousandth of a millimeter (about 0.000039 inch), is pluralized as either *micra* or *microns*.

OS

The Latin *os* in a medical context can mean either a bone or a mouth (opening). The plurals of these words are *ossa* for bones (in both English and Latin) and *ora* for mouths or openings (in both English and Latin). The genitive (possessive) case of *os*, bone, is *ossis*; the genitive of *os*, mouth, is *oris*.

The derivations are numerous: for bone, osseous, osseocartilaginous, ossify, osteoporosis; for mouth, oral, perioral, osculatory, orifice, orality.

PHENOMENON

The plural of *phenomenon* is *phenomena*. A problem arises when the writer or editor who hasn't had the benefit of a classical education confuses Latin and Greek and pluralizes every Latin- or Greek-sounding word by adding *a* or *i*. Sometimes that works and sometimes it doesn't. You could look it up.

PROPER NOUNS

Is the plural of Maple Leaf "Maple Leaves" or "Maple Leafs"? The rule here is that the plurals of proper nouns—the name of an ice hockey team in this instance—are usually made by simply adding *s* or *es*. So the members of this Canadian team are *Maple Leafs*.

Members of the Jones family are the Joneses, and members of the Heinz family are the Heinzes.

The plural of Mercedes-Benz is Mercedes-Benzes. The plural of Mercedes is Mercedeses. If you feel queasy about using this correct plural, you can always say "Mercedes-Benz vehicles." The Mercedes part comes from the first name of the daughter of Emil Jellinek, an Austrian auto-maker who liked to name his cars (three racing cars among them) for her. He talked the Daimler company into designing a car for him, which he promptly dubbed "Mercedes." When the Daimler and Benz companies merged in 1926, they kept that name.

VISCERA

Is *viscera* singular or plural? It's plural; the singular is *viscus*, which means an internal organ in both English and Latin, despite a statement I've seen that there is no singular.

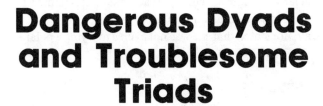

Dangerous Dyads and Troublesome Triads

Homonyms, homographs, and homophones cause much confusion in everyday speech and writing. In medical writing and editing, this bewilderment could have serious consequences.

Homophones are words that are pronounced the same but have different derivations or spellings:

> might, mite
> all, awl
> write, rite, right

Homonyms and *homographs* (the terms are virtually synonymous) are words that are spelled alike but have different meanings, derivations, or pronunciations: for example, *conduct* and *invalid*, whose meanings differ with the pronunciation.

The first element in each of these three word categories comes from the Greek *homos*, which means same. *Homonym*, from the Latin *homonymum*, means the same word used to denote different things and is from the Greek *homonymon*, a form of *homonymos*, having the same name. *Homophone* is from the International Scientific Vocabulary (ISV) *hom-* plus the Greek word for sound, voice, or tone. *Homograph* is from *hom-* plus the Greek word for writing or written.

The first element, *homo-*, in these words should not be confused with the root *hom-* or *homo-* in words or phrases such as hominoid, homocentric, hominid, *homo sapiens*, or *homo faber*, which stem from the Latin *homo*, meaning man or, sometimes, human being.

Heter- and *hetero-* are from Greek and are combining forms (usually prefixes). They mean other than or different.

Homosexual is derived from terms meaning of or relating to the same sex or to homosexuality. It is the antonym of *heterosexual*.

Other pairs or triplets, soundalikes or lookalikes not necessarily homophones, homonyms, or homographs, can be equally troublesome.

DANGEROUS DYADS AND TROUBLESOME TRIADS **105**

ADVERSE, AVERSE

Adverse means unfavorable. *Averse* means disinclined.

> Adverse criticism can be constructive as well as destructive.
> Physicians are requested to report adverse effects to the FDA.
> The rats soon became averse to the sugar water.
> The aviator stated that she was not averse to trying a polar circumnavigation again.

AFFECT, EFFECT

These words can be either nouns or verbs, and that's what causes the difficulty. *Affect* as a verb seldom causes trouble except when the writer is not sure of the spelling. Let's straighten the whole thing out.

Affect as a noun is stressed on the first syllable. It has to do with emotion or range of emotions and is rarely used except in psychology and psychiatry.

Affect as a verb (accented on the second syllable) means to have an influence or effect on something. *Effect*, which regrettably sounds and looks so much like *affect*, as a verb means to execute or accomplish.

> Too low a blood glucose level can affect the functioning of the brain, causing seizures, coma, or death.
> To effect a change in attitude, the therapist may try effecting a change also in the life situation.

If a mnemonic association is needed, the following verb forms, although not synonymous, may help:

> To *a*ffect is to *a*lter or *a*ct on.
> To *e*ffect is to *e*xecute.
> To be *e*ffective is to be *e*fficient [or, for those of us who work with pharmaceuticals, *e*fficacious (which only means effective anyway)].

For the nouns, try these mnemonic aids:

> Fl*a*t *a*ffect
> *E*nd *e*ffect

Digression on the word *mnemonic*: There are just a few words in the English language that begin with *mn*, and most of them are related to *mnemonic*. The origin of these words is the Greek term for memory. One of the Titans (Elder Gods in Greek mythology) was Mnemosyne, the goddess of memory. The nine Muses were the daughters of Zeus and Mnemosyne.

This root also appears in words such as *amnesia* and *amnesty*.

ALTERNATE, ALTERNATIVE

Although these two words are often used synonymously, the nuance of difference should be observed for the sake of clarity.

Alternate and its derivatives denote "by turns" or "in succession."

> The two paramedics performed cardiopulmonary resuscitation (CPR) alternately until the ambulance reached the emergency department.

Alternative and its derivatives denote choices rather than turns.

> Oncologists sometimes use radiation therapy and chemotherapy as an alternative or an adjunct to surgery.

ANESTHESIA, ANESTHETIC

These terms are not interchangeable. *Anesthetics* are substances or drugs used primarily to induce *anesthesia*, which is the loss of the sensation of pain, sometimes progressing to unconsciousness.

Some *anesthetics* are merely palliatives; others are more potent and can be used to effect unconsciousness just before and during surgery.

> The stage of anesthesia may be one that is "next door to death." Indeed, this profundity is usually more desirable than a shallow state.

APPRISE, APPRAISE

Apprise is seldom used incorrectly, but *appraise* is often mistakenly used when *apprise* is called for. To apprise is to inform; to appraise is to evaluate.

> Senator James asked the Secretary to keep him apprised of the department's action.
> To appraise the clinical situation accurately, one must first know the patient's history.

BEMUSED, AMUSED

"He was more bemused than bewildered by the sudden turn of events." This sentence, from an article in a respected magazine, is truly bemusing, since bemused means dazed, confused, or bewildered, *not* amused.

> Children are always amused by the penguins at the zoo.
> In *Die Fledermaus*, the besotted, nonsinging jailer is bemused by the tenor's switch in identity.

BI-, SEMI-

Some dictionaries give credence to the use of *biweekly* to mean "twice a week" in addition to or instead of "every other week."

Bi- means "two," exactly what it means in Latin, from which we get these kinds of words. This *bi-*, by the by, is not to be confused with the prefix *bio-* or its variant *bi-*, which are from the Greek *bios*, meaning life. The Middle English *bi-* is akin to the Old English *twi-*, with whose ramifications we are familiar: *twice, twilight, twin, twill* (a fabric having a double thread).

Biennium means, in both English and Latin, a period of two years; it's from *bi-*, two, and *-ennium*, from *annus*, year.

Webster III does point out in its definition that the usage of *bi-* to mean occurring two times is "often disapproved in this sense because of the likelihood of confusion" with the sense of lasting, coming, or occurring every two (*biennial*, every two years; *bimonthly*, every two months; *biweekly*, every two weeks). The entry then recommends that the reader compare *semi-*.

Here is a prime example of the mystification engendered by a descriptive dictionary, which records definitions according to frequency of use. The reader is left to wonder which is the good usage of a word. That's why books on usage are written, to be accorded a place of honor on the library shelves of good writers and editors alongside the dictionaries.

Because of the dictionaries' sanction of *bi-* to mean twice (a week, month, year) and the possibility of a serious error, the writer must be queried as to whether *biweekly* means twice a week or every other week.

Holders of subscriptions should not have to guess; the publication frequency should be spelled out clearly.

"*Ut quod ali cibus est aliis fuat acre venenum.* What's one man's poison, signor,/Is another's meat or drink" (Beaumont and Fletcher, *Love's Cure*, 1647).

CAPITAL, CAPITOL

A *capital* is the seat of government, usually of a state or a country. A *capitol* is the building in which a legislative body sits, in most instances a statehouse. And then, of course, there is our magnificent Capitol in Washington, D.C.

The word *capitol* is directly from the Latin *Capitolium*, the temple of Jupiter on the Capitoline Hill in Rome. *Capital*, also from Latin, has its root in *caput*, head.

CASUALNESS, CASUALTY

Readers of this book are undoubtedly too conversant with words and usage to confuse this dyad. However, we must think of future generations. Will the time come when young people will confuse *casualty* with *casualness*? Before you answer too quickly that this is an unlikely case, consider the marquee of a theater on which *adultery* was used to mean adulthood.

Adultery has no relation to *adult*. *Adult* is from the Latin *adultus*, the past participle of *adolescere*, to grow up. The present participle is *adolescens* (*adulescens*). *Adultery* is from the past participle of the Latin *adulterare*, to defile, pollute, or commit adultery, and ultimately from *alter*, meaning different or other.

Will the new premier of a country be confused with a master carpenter because the headline contains the word *cabinetmaker*?

COHORT, COLLEAGUE

One may be a member of a *cohort*, but other members of the group are *colleagues*, not cohorts. A cohort is a specific, discrete group or subgroup, not an individual.

> As the head psychologist, she participated in the research on a cohort consisting of adolescents.

In ancient times a cohort was one of 10 divisions of a Roman legion; each cohort comprised 300 soldiers (later increased to 500 or 600). *Cohort* and *court* (enclosure) come from the Latin *cohors* (combining form, *cohort-*) meaning enclosure or cohort.

COMPLEMENT, COMPLIMENT

A *compliment* is rarely seen in a medical or pharmaceutical context. *Compliment*, when *complement* is meant, is seen often in advertisements.

If a mnemonic aid is needed, a *complement* is a first cousin (perhaps even a sibling) to a *supplement*. The origin of *complement* is Middle English, from the Latin *complementum* and *complere*, to complete or fill up.

> This package contains complementary product samples.

The samples were free, so the sentence should have contained "complimentary," or, better yet, "free" samples.

Compliment itself, meaning a favorable, laudatory, or pleasing declaration or expression, is rarely misspelled *complement*. *Compliment* is French, from the Italian *complimento* and the Spanish *cumplimiento*, and ultimately from the Latin *cumplir* and, again, *complere*. The idea is to complete or accomplish what is due, that is, to be courteous.

> The information in this pamphlet is intended only to compliment the advice and guidance of your physician, not to replace it.

Incorrect. The information is meant to *complement*, or add to, the advice.

COMPRISE, COMPOSE

In one sense, to *compose* is to put things together—musical compositions, essays, galleys, pages. This verb is often used in the passive voice.

> A culture is composed of diverse elements.

Comprise is never used correctly in the passive voice.

> The National Institutes of Health complex comprises [*not* is comprised of] 13 institutes and several other divisions.

To put it succinctly, the parts *compose* the whole; the whole *comprises* the parts.

To *comprise* is to enclose, include, or embrace. However, although one may be embraced, one cannot be comprised.

CONVINCE, PERSUADE

Both of these words mean to sway opinion, but they are not synonymous. To *convince* is to get someone to believe something or to change a viewpoint. It is usually followed by *that*.

> The impresario convinced her that there was no claque in the audience.

To *persuade* is to get someone to do something, and is therefore usually followed by an infinitive:

> He finally persuaded the diva to take another bow.

COPYWRITE, COPYRIGHT

He who writes copy is a *copywriter*, a writer of advertising or publicity copy. She who writes plays is a playwright. She is engaged in playwriting, not playwrighting (an erroneous verb form).

One problem is that *wright* is a noun, someone who makes something; it cannot be used as a verb. *Write* and *wright* are not related at all.

Wright comes from Old Frisian and Old English words having to do with work and workers. Many names of British origin denote occupation: *Cartwright, Boatwright, Wheelwright.*

A *copyright* in the writing and publishing fields is a legal right to publish, reproduce, or dramatize a work. It would therefore be incorrect to refer to a "copywritten story in the *Wall Street Journal*." The reporter should have used *copyrighted*. The past tense of the verb *copyright* is *copyrighted*, not "copyright" or "copywrote."

> Copyrighted by the author

In the copyright line of a publication, the spelled-out *copyright* is a noun, so that "copyright © by . . ." is syntactically correct.

CORD, CHORD

"The Lost Chord," by Sir Arthur Sullivan, refers to music. In fact, *chords* do refer mainly to music, but a chord can also be a straight line joining two points on a curve.

Because of a subliminal association with music, these two terms are often confused. There is no such thing as a "vocal chord" except, perhaps, as a medical anomaly; the human voice can ordinarily reproduce only one tone at a time. What is meant is a *vocal cord*—an anatomic part.

Another *cord* is often misspelled.

> Studies are being conducted for the Veterans Administration on spinal chord injuries.

Make that *spinal cord*. Like the vocal cord, it is an anatomic part.

DEFUSE, DIFFUSE

Defuse has become fashionable in this, the era of the terrorist. Because of the similarity in pronunciation, these words are almost always written or spoken interchangeably and, therefore, incorrectly.

To *diffuse* is to disperse or scatter.

> Some gases can be diffused by aerosolization.

To *defuse* is to remove the detonator from a bomb or to eliminate an irritant.

> The model hospital administrator can defuse a nasty situation diplomatically.

Fuse comes from the Italian *fuso* and Latin *fusus*, spindle; one thinks of a dynamite fuse, which is a continuous line of explosive sheathed in a flexible cable.

DIPLOMAT, DIPLOMATE

Not all *diplomates* are tactful.

In one newspaper obituary, the deceased was referred to as a "diplomat of the American Board of Pediatrics."

Both words ultimately have the same etymology. They come from the Latin *diploma*, a passport or document conferring a privilege or honor, and from the Greek *diploma*, also meaning a passport or a folded or doubled-over paper (Greek *diploos*, double).

A *diplomate* is one holding a diploma, a "document granted by a competent authority [especially a university or college] conferring some honour, privilege, or licence" (*Oxford English Dictionary, OED*). A *diplomat*, usually a government official—unless one is referring to an average citizen who is tactful or discreet—also holds a diploma of sorts. Originally a diploma (the "folded paper") was a state letter of recommendation; later it became a letter of license or privilege, thus a credential. *Diploma* is a back formation from French *diplomatique* (after, *par exemple, aristocrate, aristocratique*).

The writer of the obituary should have referred to that physician as a *diplomate*; editorializing is best left to the editorial page or the Op-Ed columns.

DISCREET, DISCRETE

These two words are often mistaken one for the other; sometimes a typist assumes that *discrete* must be a typographic error.

The lesions of smallpox are discrete (distinct).
Human traits are not discrete, like sticks in a bundle, but interact.
Gases are made up of discrete units, that is, molecules.
A discreet (tactful) silence followed her companion's faux pas.
To be discreet is to be circumspect.
The discreet way is the judicious way.

Both words are from the same Latin root, *discretus*, the past participle of *discernere*, to discern, separate, or distinguish. *Discreteness* refers to separateness, distinction, unrelatedness. *Discretion* refers to the possession of good judgment—discernment, tactfulness, prudence—in conduct, especially in speech.

DISINTERESTED, UNINTERESTED

Disinterested means impartial, unbiased, neutral. *Uninterested* means apathetic, indifferent, simply not interested.

If I were an attorney, I wouldn't under any circumstances want to appear before an *uninterested* judge, but I certainly would want her or him to be *disinterested.*

The distinction between these two words should be preserved. The antonym of *disinterested* is *interested*, which implies that something is at stake, as in an *interested party* or a *conflict of interest.*

One difficulty arises in misunderstanding of the prefixes. *Un-* is a negative prefix and is usually passive; *dis-*, also a negative prefix, is usually active. If one is uninclined, one merely has a lack of inclination; however, if one is disinclined, one has an inclination *against. Uninterested* is an achromatic word; *disinterested* is a dynamic word, denoting freedom from a personal motive.

DOSE, DOSAGE

These words are not synonymous or interchangeable, although in general they both have to do with medication or radiation.

A *dose* is the quantity administered at one time or the total quantity administered. The *dosage* is the regulation or frequency of doses.

Therefore, *dose* could be thought of as a one-shot deal, and *dosage* as the timing or periodicity.

Dosage is just about the same as *regimen*, so "dosage regimen" is redundant.

> The medication should be given in divided doses until the fever subsides.
>
> A specialist in radiation therapy and nuclear medicine can determine the correct dose of radiation.
>
> The ideal dosage is the minimum dose and frequency of daily administration that will prevent paroxysmal tachycardia.

The word *dose* is from the French *dose* and the Late Latin *dosis* and, ultimately, from a Greek word meaning the act of giving.

EFFECTIVENESS, EFFICACY

These words are virtually synonymous and interchangeable. Drugs that are *effective* are *efficacious*; the latter simply sounds more elegant but may be considered pretentious by some.

ENORMITY, IMMENSITY

If size is the sole consideration, forget *enormity.* This word refers not to great size but to outrageousness, heinousness, monstrousness. If great size is meant, *hugeness, massiveness,* or *immensity* would be correct.

The enormity of the crime led the jury to convict the defendant.

Immensity is always relative—it depends on whether you're an astronaut or an ant.

Strunk and White define *enormity* as "monstrous wickedness."

FEWER, LESS

Fewer, which is rarely misused, is correct for individuals or units of any kind:

The hazards of smoking are fewer if the smoker finally quits.

Fewer than seven members will not constitute a quorum.

There are fewer side effects with this medication, but there it is less effective.

Less, which is often mistakenly used interchangeably with *fewer*, is correct for mass or quantity, and is sometimes used with plurals when the meaning is actually quantity rather than units.

There is less heroism in refusing to dare than in daring and failing.

The odds against admission to that university may be less when the applicant is from out of state.

The Rockies are less than 45 miles from that city.

Their entire yearly budget was less than a million dollars.

Following this logic, it would be proper to write, "A million dollars has been allocated for this project," since one thinks of a million dollars as a unit, not as a million separate dollars.

FLAMMABLE, INFLAMMABLE

These words come from the Latin *flammare*, to set on fire, and they both mean "capable of being easily ignited."

When next you see a huge tanker truck rumble by with "flammable" plastered across the back, be sure to keep at least two car lengths behind.

Why *flammable* now and not the heretofore invariable *inflammable*? The former has been preferred to the latter for the past 25 years or so, especially in a technical context.

Theodore M. Bernstein wrote of "nonphilologists in the population" who may learn philology the hard way by mishandling a can of cleaning fluid labeled "inflammable." These people, he said, never give a thought to other meanings of the prefix *in-*, as in *incarcerate*, *incise*, or *inflame*. Nevertheless, he added, "if it will save a single burned eyelash, by all means let's have *flammable* . . ."

One question: Would a demagogue *flame* a mob?

FLAUNT, FLOUT

To *flout* is to have contempt for, to defy; to *flaunt* is to show ostentatiously or show off.

> They flaunted their newly acquired degrees like banners.
> He has not deliberately flouted the Hippocratic oath.

FOR EXAMPLE, THAT IS

The phrase *that is* introduces a definition and is used to reinforce what precedes it; it is specific. *For example* sets forth illustrations or examples.

> When antidepressants are used, another group of drugs, that is, diuretics, is contraindicated.
> If you are taking penicillin G by mouth, wait one hour before drinking acidic fruit juices, for example, orange or grapefruit juice.

Exempli gratia (which means for instance or for [the sake of] example), abbreviated *e.g.*, and *id est* (that is), abbreviated *i.e.*, are not interchangeable. These Latin phrases are far apart in meaning:

> The ecologist stated that the world environment is threatened by the "hothouse effect," i.e. [that is to say] [not e.g. or for example], destruction of the earth's ozone layer.
> The responsibility of the group leader is to explain the alternatives, for example [e.g.], substitution of biodegradable products for plastic ones.

Many writers prefer to use the English equivalents.

FORTUITOUS, FORTUNATE

If grammarians could bank a dollar for each misuse of *fortuitous*, they would all be rich.

Fortunate, originally from the Latin *fortuna*, is not synonymous with *fortuitous*.

> Many researchers are fortunate enough to receive federal grants.

Fortuitous, from the Latin *forte* (by chance), the ablative case of *fors* (chance), means accidental.

> The fortuitous overdose of a prescribed drug caused the death of this celebrated actress.

Writers who want to be really fancy should try *aleatoric*. This word, which means chancy or random, refers to a certain kind of music and other endeavors as well. It comes from the Latin *alea*, a game of hazard or dice. Suetonius asserted that when Caesar's troops crossed the Rubicon, the emperor-general exclaimed, "*Iacta alea est!*" ("The die is cast".)

> Innumerate people are not aware of the aleatoric aspects of our lives.

GANTLET, GAUNTLET

Although *gantlet* is a variant of *gauntlet* etymologically speaking, the one without a *u* is usually limited to parallel lines (of people or of railroad tracks) and is sometimes used in a figurative sense.

A *gauntlet* is a glove, and is almost always used in the phrase "to throw down the gauntlet," meaning to challenge.

> Fortunately, the hazing was mild—the initiate had to run through a gantlet, two lines of upperclassmen, each brandishing a stick.
>
> The originator of that genetic technique thereby threw the gauntlet down to other cancer researchers.

One kind of *gantlet* is a stretch of railroad track where two separate lines are briefly overlapped, with one rail of each track within the rails of another, so that switching becomes unnecessary.

GENDER, SEX

Sex is seldom misused, except when "to have sex" is used colloquially to mean "to have sexual intercourse." Despite popular usage, *sex* pertains to anatomic, biologic, and physiologic characteristics, not the act of sexual intercourse.

To avoid repetition, to appear fastidious, or to make a point, some writers use the word *gender* interchangeably with *sex*. In disciplines such as psychology, psychiatry, and sexology, *gender* is sometimes used to denote psychologic aspects in contrast to purely physiologic characteristics.

> Words in certain languages undergo changes as an indication of gender, number, tense, and so on.
>
> The insurance industry tends to ignore sex in calculating automobile insurance premiums.

In some other languages, for example, French, gender is assigned arbitrarily without regard to true sex, if any. In Latin most words ending in *-a* are feminine in gender; however, *agricola*, farmer, is masculine in gender. English has common gender—a real time-saver for impatient Americans.

Gender, a ubiquitous term in the writings of language experts, refers to words. The *New York Times* "bulletin of second-guessing," *Winners & Sinners*, says that "words have gender. People, bless their hearts, have sex."

HANGED, HUNG

> Police said it appeared that he had hanged himself.
>
> In some states, people who are convicted of capital crimes are hanged.
>
> The stockings were hung by the chimney with care.

In short, people are *hanged*; things are *hung*.

HONE, HOME

To *hone* is to use a stone or other method to sharpen something, such as a razor or a skill.

> Oliver Wendell Holmes's wit was honed to as sharp an edge as his scalpel.
>
> To paraphrase Washington Irving, the tongue is the only edged tool that grows sharper with the honing of constant use.

Homing is returning to a specific location or reaching a specific target and is usually followed by *in* or *on*.

> Salmon always home in on the same spawning grounds.
>
> Swallows home in on San Juan Capistrano every March 19 and leave about October 23.
>
> It was not until a few years ago that scientists began to home in on the oncogene.
>
> The problem was to have the laser home in on the plaque without harming the healthy tissue.

The homing pigeon is not to be confused with the humming pigeon or the hummingbird.

ILEUM, ILEUS

The *ileum* (in Latin and English) is the last part of the small intestine, between the jejunum and the large intestine.

Ileus, the Latin twin of the Greek *eileos* (from *eilein*, to roll up), is a potentially dire obstruction of the intestines.

Look out for typographic errors! They can be lethal.

IMPLY, INFER

These two words cause a great deal of trouble in conversation, since it is often difficult to think of the right word and meaning on the spur of the moment.

To *imply* is to speak indirectly or to suggest. To *infer* is to surmise or conclude.

> Are you implying that surgery is a practical alternative?
>
> I infer from your statement that you agree with my solution to this difficult problem.

Theodore Bernstein came up with this sporty mnemonic association: to think of the one who implies as the pitcher and the one who infers as the catcher.

Another association is to visualize the relation between printer's type and paper: The first (the implier) delivers an impression, and the second (the inferrer) accepts it.

INCIDENCE, PREVALENCE

Incidence is the rate of occurrence or the amount or extent of an occurrence, for example, the number of new cases of a particular disease occurring during a particular period of time. Incidence reports a rate and is expressed as occurrences per unit time.

Prevalence is the total number (or percentage) of cases of a particular disease or disorder existing at a certain time in a certain area, or the state of being widespread, common, or prevailing.

No doubt epidemiologists, statisticians, and other scientists and researchers would be grateful to see these technical terms used accurately and appropriately.

> The incidence of acute myocardial infarction in men was fewer than 3 for every 1,000 over a 7-year period.
>
> On Monday the prevalence of pneumonia in the surgical suites was 6%.

Incidence expresses the number of new cases. *Prevalence* expresses the total number of cases; it is usually used when time is not a crucial factor in the results and when the results represent a proportion of a discrete population or cohort.

INSTALLATION, INSTILLATION

These words should not be confused, especially in a medical or pharmaceutical context.

> The nursing staff awaited the installation of the new device.
>
> The physician prescribed instillation of this medication for the greatest effectiveness.

Instillation is from the Latin *instillare*—from *stillare*, meaning to trickle or drip.

Installation is directly from the Latin *installare*, meaning to install. An installation can be possession or conferring of an office or a setting up of equipment.

INTER-, INTRA-

Early in the collaboration between writer and word processor operator, if they be twain and not ain, the w.p.o. should be instructed to be painstakingly accurate in typing *inter-* and *intra-*.

Intraocular (within the eye) is vastly different from *interocular* (located between the eyes).

The *interventricular* septum is a wall between ventricles; there is no such thing as an intraventricular septum, but there can be an *intraventricular* (within a ventricle) condition.

INTERMENT, INTERNMENT

These are actual newspaper excerpts:

> She will be interned at the Golden Gate National Cemetery.

> The Commissioner of Immigration and Naturalization had "selectively interred" 10,000 Italians and Germans on the East Coast as "potentially dangerous" during the war.

Interment, being burial, is not a laughing matter. Neither was or is *internment*, which is incarceration, or imprisonment.

By the way, an incarcerated hernia is constricted but not strangulated.

INVERSE, REVERSE, OBVERSE, CONVERSE

Does this questionable quartet create a quandary?

Inverse means directly opposite. *Reverse* means with the back presented. *Obverse* means facing the front of the observer or opponent. *Converse* means about the same as inverse—opposite.

These words all have the same root: the Latin verb *vertere*, to turn.

LITERALLY, FIGURATIVELY

> He was literally dying to get into that particular medical college.

Too bad. He would have made a fine physician.

Literally means actually, in fact, de facto, verbatim, no kidding, and without metaphor or exaggeration.

Figuratively means metaphorically or as a figure of speech.

Don't take either her praise or her criticism too *literally*.

Thoreau was speaking *figuratively* when he referred to his lake as a "thread of finest gossamer stretched across the valley."

MASTERLY, MASTERFUL

Masterly is rarely if ever misused and *masterful* is almost always misused. One reason might be that *masterly* makes an awkward (although technically correct) adverb and *masterfully* an exceedingly expressive one.

Masterly means in the manner of a master or an artist:

Her command of English was masterly even though it was her second language.

Masterful means overbearing, arrogant, domineering:

MacArthur addressed his troops in his customary masterful manner.

It might help to remember that *-ly* means "like"; it comes from a Germanic term embodying that meaning.

If "he directed the motion picture masterly" grates on your ear, try something like "he directed the motion picture in a masterly [or artistic] manner."

MEAN, MEDIAN, AVERAGE

Mean and *median* are statistical terms; *average* is sometimes statistical also.

The *mean* is a type of average. One can find the arithmetic mean of a group of numbers by dividing the sum by the number of members in the group. For example, the sum of the seven numbers 4, 5, 6, 9, 13, 14, and 19 is 70, so their mean is 70 divided by 7, or 10. The mean here is synonymous with the average.

The *median* is another type of average. In a group of numbers, there are as many numbers of the group that are larger than the median as there are smaller. In the group 4, 5, 6, 9, 13, 14, and 19, the median is 9, because three numbers are larger and three are smaller. When there is an even number of numbers in the group, the median is usually defined as the number halfway between the middle pair.

The *average* pay of five workers earning $10, $14, $20, $26, and $40 a day is $22, but the median is only $20, because there are two workers above and two below that figure.

MEDICATION, MEDICINE, MEDICAMENT

These words are virtually synonymous; they can all mean therapeutic preparations or drugs.

Medication, without the article *a*, can also mean the treatment itself or administration of a therapeutic preparation.

Medicine can also be defined as the science and art of maintaining health and preventing disease, or a branch of medicine (sometimes called internal medicine) dealing with nonsurgical treatment, and as differentiated from obstetrics and surgery. It can be used figuratively: "Laughter is good medicine."

MILITATE, MITIGATE

Militate, from the Latin *militatus*, a form of the word for soldier, means to have weight or effect and is almost always followed by *against*.

> This situation results from fiscal pressures that militate against hospitalizing patients for what the agency might consider outpatient procedures.

Mitigate, from the Latin *mitigare* (to soften or mitigate), means to extenuate, soften, temper, lessen, palliate.

> Drug addicts use these substances to mitigate the hardships they perceive as insoluble.

Mitigate is never followed by *against*.

MULTIFACTORIAL, MULTIFACTORAL

There is little occasion in writing to use the word *multifactorial* except in the world of genetics. After having seen this term misused over the years to mean "having many factors," I minted the word *multifactoral*. So far my coinage has not made it into the dictionaries.

NAUSEOUS, NAUSEATED

To be *nauseous* is to cause nausea, to be loathsome or abhorrent. To be *nauseated* is to become ill. The *-ous* in *nauseous* has the same effect as in *poisonous*.

> Emetics are meant to be *nauseous*, so that people can be purged of toxic substances.
>
> The inhabitants of certain cities in the eastern corridor are sometimes *nauseated* by severe air pollution.

The English word *nausea* is the same as the Latin; it means, literally, seasickness, and comes from the Greek word for ship.

This distinction should be preserved, especially by those who are educated and informed, and certainly by medical writers and editors.

NORMAL, ORDINARY

In everyday usage, it makes little difference whether *normal* is used synonymously with *ordinary*. However, in medical writing and editing this differentiation is sometimes blurred.

It is good practice to substitute *ordinary* for *normal* when the meaning is "usual" or "routine," and to confine the use of *normal* to mean the opposite of *abnormal*. "In normal circumstances" may mean something entirely different from "in ordinary circumstances."

For more on *normal,* see the entry on "Abnormal, normal" in Chapter 15, "Jargon: Medicalese, Journalese, Professionalese," under "Medicalese."

OS, OS

These two words are hardly ever confused, since one means "bone" and the other means "mouth"or "orifice." The context will almost certainly be unambiguous.

A fuller treatment of these terms is given in Chapter 11, "Singular Plurals." See also "Verbal, oral" in this chapter.

-OTOMY, -OSTOMY

When the writer means a cutting out, cutting off, or cutting into, with the opening or the incision to be closed at the end of the operation, the suffix *-otomy* should be used.

> Because the patient was exsanguinating rapidly, the surgeons performed a vagotomy and pyloroplasty.

In that sentence, *vagotomy* refers to a selective cutting (through) of the vagus nerve at the site of the patient's duodenal ulcer to remedy excessive secretion of acid.

The suffix *-ostomy* denotes the surgical formation of an opening or mouth, usually retained permanently or for a definite or specified time.

> The newborn infant's life was saved by a gastrostomy.

PARENTAL, PARENTERAL

Three letters make all the difference between a *parental* feeding and a *parenteral* feeding.

If a father or mother does the honors, it's *parental*. If the feeding or nutrition is *parenteral*, it's not in or through the digestive system—it's feeding or the administration of nutrients intradermally, intramuscularly, intravenously, or subcutaneously. They do not provide complete nutrition, but parenteral fluids, usually physiologic saline solutions, are used to maintain patients' electrolyte balance after surgery and in conditions such as shock, malnutrition, malabsorption, coma, and hepatic and renal failure.

PHOSPHORUS, PHOSPHOROUS

Phosphorus is an element of the nitrogen family and is a noun. The word *phosphorous* is an adjective and means phosphorescent, sometimes used to describe waves at night. *Phosphorous* is also used to describe a compound in which phosphorus has a valence lower than in phosphoric compounds.

When it stands alone, and in lists of blood chemistry values, it should always be *phosphorus, not phosphorous.*

> The resolution of low-energy phosphorous signals is an important limitation for which no solution has yet been found.

Even in light of the context, it is difficult to know whether the writer meant "phosphorus signals" or "signals resembling those made by phosphorus." The writer must be queried.

PORE, POUR

> The demographers poured over the information for weeks.

What was meant here was *pored*, meaning that they read the information carefully and attentively. Apparently it's the "over" that confuses some writers.

> Statisticians had to carefully pour over the records to uncover the additional deaths.

Since this seemed a serious occasion, champagne was not poured. The editor must have been out to launch.

PRECIPITOUS, PRECIPITATE

Precipitous is always an adjective; it means steep (either up or down). *Precipitate* as an adjective means hasty, rash, abrupt.

> The percentage of the budget spent on administration has dropped precipitously.
>
> There is no record that such precipitate action was taken in violation of medical and ethical conduct and practice.

To keep the distinction in mind, you might try associating the *s* in *s*teep with precipitou*s*, and the *a* in *a*brupt with precipit*a*te.

PRESCRIBED, PROSCRIBED

To *prescribe* is to direct, lay down rules, or give or write a prescription for someone.

> In college you will be forced into a prescribed curriculum with limited choices.
>
> The internist prescribed a newly approved orphan drug for the patient's seizures.
>
> *Robert's Rules of Order* prescribes the sequence of a motion.

To *proscribe* is to forbid, prohibit, condemn:

> Many states proscribe the death penalty for capital crimes.
>
> Why should the use of European-approved drugs be proscribed in this instance?

PRINCIPAL, PRINCIPLE

Both words originate in the Latin *princeps*, which means chief or first person (as a noun) and first (as an adjective). *Princeps* is synthesized from a form of the Latin *primus*, first (*prin-*) plus a form of *capio* (*capere*, to take). *Principal* can be either a noun or an adjective; *principle* is always a noun.

> As the principal of the school [noun], she was responsible for its curricula. (Mnemonic aid: The princi*pal* is a *pal*.)
>
> Dr. Enos Iznaim was the principal investigator [adjective] in this clinical trial.

Here is an incorrect use:

> With the medical profession on the attack, heart disease, the principle killer of Americans, may soon be in retreat.

Heart disease kills people—not principles. Statistics tell us that more people die of accidental deaths, but heart disease remains the principal (main, chief, most significant, most consequential, most important) killer when it comes to natural deaths.

This magnificent excerpt from a legal opinion illustrates the correct use of the word *principle*:

> If there is any principle of the Constitution that more imperatively calls for attachment than any other it is the principle of free thought—not free thought for those who agree with us but freedom for the thought that we hate.

This opinion was written in *United States* v. *Schwimmer*, 279 U.S. 644,653 (1928), by the wise and justly famous Oliver Wendell Holmes (1841–1935), son of the equally illustrious Oliver Wendell Holmes, M.D. (1809–1894).

The junior Holmes, after service in the Union army in the Civil War, was admitted to the bar in 1867. He became a professor of law at the Harvard Law School, and later chief justice of the Massachusetts Supreme Court. In 1902 he was appointed associate justice of the United States Supreme Court, on which he served for 30 years.

Some of his opinions were so perspicuous and elegantly written that they were published as *The Dissenting Opinions of Mr. Justice Holmes* in 1929.

PRONE, SUPINE

These two words have opposite meanings. To be *prone* is to lie with one's face downward. To be *supine* is to lie on one's back, with the face upward.

> Because the patient's spine was fractured, he was brought into the trauma emergency room prone.
>
> For laparotomy and certain other surgical operations, patients are supine on the operating table.

REGIME, REGIMEN

These words are from the Latin *regimen*, a directing, guiding, or controlling.

Regime, however, is usually confined to the idea of ruling or guiding (a country, for instance) for a specific time.

A *regimen* is a systematic or planned guidance, as in a diet or medication regimen.

RESTIVE, RESTLESS

The first four letters are the same, but these words are far from interchangeable or synonymous.

Restless means constantly moving, uneasy, unquiet.

Psychotic patients are sometimes restless and hebephrenic.

Restive, from the Middle English *restife* (meaning stationary, as spoken of animals), means balky, obstinate, unmoving. *Restife* is ultimately from the French *rester*, to remain or stay behind.

Three riders in the Grand Canyon were thrown by restive burros.

People, of course, can also be restive.

RETICENT, RELUCTANT

The aged rats especially were reticent to enter the treadmill.

They weren't *reticent*—they were *reluctant*. I can't say I blame them.

The AIDS virus is reticent to therapy.

Resistant or refractory—not *reticent*.

Reticent does not mean reluctant, hesitant, or resistant. Here its etymology is the clue. It comes from the Latin *reticere*, to be silent or quiet. A reticent person is one who keeps silent in the supermarket when someone steps in front of her in the checkout line.

Harpo (né Adolph or Arthur) Marx was the ultimate in reticent people. He spoke only with his ever-present bicycle horn. His *nom cinématique* was more apt than perhaps even he, with his unpublicized intellectual attainments, might have known.

The harp he played so ravishingly was the reason for his name. Another that occurs to me is the name in Roman mythology for the Egyptian god Horus as a boy—Harpocrates. This god was invariably pictured with his finger to his lips to enjoin discreet silence. Cupid had bribed Harpocrates with a rose to keep Venus's amours secret.

USE, USAGE, UTILIZE

The simple word *use* is underused. *Usage* means traditional or customary practice; it pertains to mores as well as to words. It should not be used as a variant of *use*.

To utilize is to use to advantage.

Many cities are now *utilizing* trash or garbage to generate power and make fuel.

Use is strong enough to stand on its own three feet.

VERBAL, ORAL

Verbal, from the Latin word for word, *verbum,* pertains to words. There is no implicit differentiation between oral and written expressions in *verbal.*

Oral is from the Latin word for mouth or orifice, *os* (genitive case, *oris*). "Per os" ("P.O." or "p.o.") on a prescription is an instruction to take the medicine orally, by mouth. Many English words contain this root, among them *aboral, peroral,* and *oralogy* (stomatology). *Oration* is from a different Latin root, *oratio,* which means speaking, speech, language.

The plural of the anatomic term *os,* meaning mouth, is *ora.* Care should be taken to ensure that the proper plural is used, especially in a medical context. The plural of *os* (from Latin; genitive case, *ossis*) meaning bone is *ossa.* Words that contain this root include *osseous, ossicle, ossification,* and *osteoarthritis.*

Some writers are famous for their verbal virtuosity.

Verbal is used correctly in the preceding sentence, since it refers to the writers' talent for expression with words.

Wilson had reneged on a verbal contract to share the clinic's profits with her.

Most likely the contract was an oral one, a far cry from a written one although just as legal in certain circumstances.

Two of the Department of State employees had been given letters of reprimand, and the third was criticized verbally.

Criticized orally. It would be difficult to criticize in any manner other than with words, except for certain nonverbal (sometimes rude and crude) gestures.

Verbal results of the patient's tests will be called in to you the same day—followed by a written report and hard-copy images for your files.

The context indicates transmission of the results by telephone. The initial results would therefore be orally conveyed.

There is a choice between using a word that has two possible meanings, *verbal* (in words, whether spoken or written) and using a word that is more precise, *oral.* The latter should therefore be used in referring to spoken language; *verbal* is preferable in referring to written language only.

VIRAL, VIRILE

Think of it! Young, viral men are driven in golf carts from the bullpen to the mound to save time.

Virile!

This antivirile drug is still being tested for its effect on certain kinds of cancer.

A mistake like that could cause pharmaceutical stocks to plummet precipitously. *Antiviral!*

Both of these words are from Latin. *Virus* means slime, stench, or poison. *Virile*, from the Latin word for man (and perhaps ultimately from Latin *vis*, strength), is synonymous with *masculine* and means having the characteristics of an adult man.

WROUGHT, WREAKED

What hath God wreaked?

What hath God *wrought*.

Nature has wrought her vengeance on them by slowing down their metabolism.

Nature has *wreaked* her vengeance.

Wrought is an alternative past tense of *work* and now is seen mainly in connection with things that are molded, fashioned, or shaped by hand.

Wreaked means inflicted, afflicted, punished, or avenged. It is from the Middle English *wreken*, meaning drive out, punish, or avenge.

Dealers in illicit drugs can wreck havoc in a residential community.

They can—and do—wreak havoc.

Most people live their entire lives without hearing these words in conversation. Both *wrought* and *wreaked* have a faintly anachronistic but pleasant aroma.

YOKES, YOLKS

This book yolks reminiscences of the author to an argument suggesting that this particular religion be abandoned for the good of the human species.

Make that *yokes*, to obviate a superfluity of cholesterol. Some yolk, eh kid?

CHAPTER 13

Tautology

The title of this chapter is Tautology rather than Redundancy, because any *-ology* sounds much more learned. However, I could have used Superfluity, Verbosity, Verbiage, Periphrasis, or Prolixity.

Besides, there are many kinds of redundancies, but *tautology* has to do specifically with unnecessary repetition of words, ideas, or statements. *Tautology* is the keynote speaker saying, "Before I speak, I'd like to say a few words."

SOME PRIME EXAMPLES OF TAUTOLOGY

Who will be appointed to head up the agency?

What purpose does *up* serve?

Advance planning will obviate most of the difficulties.

All planning is advance. By definition, planning cannot be retroactive.

He's a handsome-looking man.

Handsome-looking is as handsome-looking does.

Her job was to teach the basic fundamentals of pharmacology.

Or the fundamental basics? The writer of that gem should look up the definition of *fundament*. (In *Webster III* it's definition 2a.)

Monday's game was attended by approximately 400 to 500 people.

Too approximate. Approximately 450 would be all right. Delete the nervous *approximately*.

Difficulties arose early on.

This sentence is even choppier if one chops off the final, redundant word, as one should. It could be recast to read: "Difficulties arose early in the investigation [or other such formulation]."

Intradermal skin tests were performed as usual.

Are there other kinds of intradermal tests?

The cells were red in color.

And the blood was blue in color.

For the ultimate in perfection . . .

Perfection *is* the ultimate.

Her face was oval-shaped.

Some people's faces are round-shaped.

This is the most unique medical center in the world.

Or the galaxy? *Unique* is an incomparable adjective, and as such cannot be modified except perhaps by "truly" or "perhaps."

We believe the potential hazards of this product are extremely minimal.

Sounds as if someone is trying to stonewall on a carcinogen. *Hazard* has *potential* built into it; *extremely* and *potential* are redundant. The meaning of *minimal*—down to the bare bones, that is, the least possible in size, number, or degree—renders the adverb *extremely* redundant.

The hospital's Board of Trustees finally reached a consensus of opinion on the new building.

Of opinion is redundant. *Consensus*, the Latin past participle of *consentire*, meaning to agree, has nothing to do with *census*, which is from the Latin *censere*, meaning to assess or tax. Now you know why censuses are taken.

The faculty cannot act until the true facts are known and made public.

Facts are by definition true. "False facts" is unthinkable. Delete *true*.

We are apprehensive about the end result of this budget cut in research.

The end is the result and the result is the end. A simple *result* will do.

We need not know the cause of a disease or disorder in order to treat it, although of course that would be invaluable information.

In order to is redundant and usually disrupts the rhythm of a sentence. Plain *to* in purposeful meaning is preferable in every instance. I have rarely seen an *in order to* that could not be reduced to a simple *to*.

It is too soon to predict the outcome of this illness based on the fact that the medication has not had time to become effective.

". . . illness, because the medication . . ." By recasting the sentence, the writer has saved several characters (about 15) and has also improved the rhythm of the sentence.

Drug supplies used in these studies were supplied by Apex International.

Supplies is redundant. "The drugs used . . . " would have been adequate.

The investigators arrived at the conclusion that focusing too hard on a video terminal all day does have deleterious effects, but that eye exercises are beneficial and effective.

Economy, economy, economy. "The investigators concluded that focusing . . ."

The erythrocyte proved to be an excellent model for the in-vitro evaluation of this syndrome.

Two things: (1) *proved to be* should read *was*; (2) in vitro, in vivo, and other such foreign terms are never hyphenated, even when they are (as in this instance) compound adjectives. Neither are they italicized. This usage differs from British usage. (See the section on "In vitro, in vivo" under "Hyphens" in Chapter 7, "Punctuation.")

She served as chief executive officer and chair of the board for 15 years.

"She was the chief executive officer . . ." is preferable.

Prior to infusion, the patient had received a corticosteroid.

"Before infusion . . ."

Subsequent to the introduction of halothane in 1956, many cases of hepatotoxicity began to be recorded.

"After the introduction . . ."

Following the collision, the injured were rushed to the medical center by helicopter.

"After the collision . . ."

In the majority of adolescent cases, AIDS was diagnosed years after these patients had received blood transfusions.

"In most adolescent cases . . ." If the nature of the *majority* is not spelled out, usually in the form of a percentage, *most* will almost always suffice.

In the majority of instances, patients seek medical advice only when their routine functioning is disturbed.

Try *ordinarily* or *usually* instead of the wordy (and sometimes imprecise) "in the majority of instances": "Patients usually seek medical advice . . ."

The long-term survivors are currently in good health.

More than half of the patients are hospitalized at the present time.

At present it is probable that the mortality will remain at the current low figure.

In each of these three sentences, the adverb or the adverbial phrase is redundant. *Currently, at the present time,* and *at present* all mean "now"; they are redundant anyhow, because the verb in each instance is in the present tense. In the last sentence, *current* is a clue in addition to the present tense *is.*

It should be noted here that *presently,* although it sounds as if it means "now," actually means "soon."

They sought an arbitrator for the purpose of circumventing the court.

"They sought an arbitrator to circumvent the court" is preferable.

The problem arose for the simple reason that the commission would not accept responsibility.

The problem arose *only because* the commission would not accept responsibility. The writer could have saved four words.

SUPERCILIOUSNESS AND CONDESCENSION

It is clear that this drug, which is now in phase III testing, will augment the leukocyte count and may be beneficial in counteracting the side effects of chemotherapy.

If it is clear, why say "it is clear"? This phrase, like "it is obvious," is supercilious and unnecessary. If a bridge (transitional phrase) is needed from one sentence to the next, try *hence* or *therefore.*

See also "Obviously, clear" in Chapter 16, "Faddy and Supercilious Words."

LEGAL LANGUAGE

The language of the law is full of redundancies. One reason is given in another chapter (see the discussion of "And/or" in Chapter 9, "Double Meanings"). However, lawyers are much given to such redundancies as *if, as, and when,* when a simple *when* would suffice. *Each and every* is another one.

Unless the author is being paid by the word, economy is the watchword.

WASP

The *W* in the acronym WASP is redundant (although the acronym is inspired), since all "Anglo-Saxon Protestants," Americans of Northern European extraction and Protestant background, are white.

This WASP, in use since 1960, is not to be confused with WASP, *W*omen's *A*ir Force *S*ervice *P*ilots, or the *W*eber *A*dvanced *S*patial *P*erception test. It is attributed to Digby Baltzell, a Philadelphia author and sociologist, who used it to characterize, not too favorably, an individual in a certain privileged class.

ECONOMY OF WORDS

Few writers could equal the feat of Watson and Crick, who described the double helix (the molecular structure of nucleic acids) in 900 words, one table, and six references. Arthur Kornberg reported on the enzymatic synthesis of DNA in 430 words. Cournand and Ranges reported on the first catheterization of the human heart in 950 words. Fritz A. Lipmann described coenzyme A in 250 words, one table, and five references. (Source for these data: Martin M. Cummings, M.D., former Director of the National Library of Medicine, in his Honor Lecture in 1973 before the American Medical Writers Association, as modified from his Sigma Xi Distinguished Lecture in 1972.)

Enough said. I don't want to be redundant, prolix, verbose, tautologic, or pleonastic.

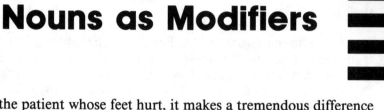

CHAPTER 14

Nouns as Modifiers

For the patient whose feet hurt, it makes a tremendous difference whether the Doctor of Podiatric Medicine is a callus remover or a callous remover.

THE VERSATILITY OF ENGLISH

English is a versatile, flexible language; its boosters will undoubtedly use these attributes in their argument for English as a world language. Nouns have been used as modifiers in English as long as the language has existed. Indeed, nouns can also be used felicitously and grammatically as parts of speech other than nouns or adjectives. One would not ordinarily say "musical critic" or "scientific editor." A music critic may or may not be musical, and a science editor may be unscientific in work habits. And does it really matter whether an editor is religious or irreligious if he or she is the religion editor?

Nonetheless, the acceptable term is "medical writer," not "medicine writer." Why? Well, it's idiomatic, an adjective that "explains" many inconsistencies in the language. An *idiom* is a structural form peculiar to a particular people or to a district, community, or class. Despite the preceding paragraph, "scientific editor" or "scientific writer" is acceptable; the phrase means merely that the editor or writer deals with scientific matters.

What about "juvenile court," "criminal lawyer," and other such seemingly ludicrous terms? Once I was asked whether there is such a person as a child psychiatrist. I can state—without fear of contradiction—that there is such a person.

Bergen Evans and Cornelia Evans (brother and sister) made the following cogent point in *A Dictionary of Contemporary American Usage*:

> Occasionally someone notices that the first element in one of these compounds can be read as an adjective. This is all very well as a source of innocent merriment. But anyone who concludes that [such a] compound is a grammatical mistake and solemnly goes about condemning it and those who use it, is being ridiculous. These words

are part of the fabric of the language and anyone who hopes to get rid of them will have to remake the language.

I doubt that anyone can substitute an adjective for the noun *labor* in "labor market" without vitiating the meaning.

The richness and versatility of English make it possible for the "same" word to be used as many different parts of speech. Here are some examples of this phenomenon:

Fast can be a noun (breaking the fast), an adjective (fast train), and an adverb (to make the Hindenburg fast). It can also be a verb (to fast before a surgical procedure).

Better can be a noun (aping their betters), a verb (to better the odds on survival), an adjective (it is a far, far better thing that I do), and an adverb (if you can do it better, do it).

While can quadruple in brass:

> Students were whiling away the time before class. (verb)
> Gather ye rosebuds while ye may. (conjunction)
> It will be worth your while to publish this finding. (noun)

Those are only three parts of speech, you say? The fourth use is archaic—from Shakespeare: "While [until] then, God be with you" (preposition).

Down and *out* can each be used as five parts of speech: noun, verb, preposition, adjective, and adverb. If you enjoy word aerobics, try them on your own.

AGGLOMERATION OF MODIFIERS

Good writers are never guilty of a mannerism termed "polymerization" or "lamination," the piling on of several adjectives or nouns to modify one lone noun. What is one to think about this ungainly example?

> The current drug comparison studies data base included 500 patients.

Attempting to achieve *multum in parvo*, the author of an article committed this titular indiscretion:

> Chlorpromazine Mild to Moderate Psychosis Progress Report No. 3.

Perhaps in an attempt to be cute, the principals of a firm announced the formation of an "equity-oriented venture capital limited partnership small business investment company."

A photograph on the cover of a medical journal displays the "1989 American Nurses' Association National Nurses' Day Poster." Here compression, dictated by space limitations, wins the day—seven words modify "poster."

A single noun shouldn't be called on to support such a burden. Wilson Follett deplored the "agglutination of ideas into complex phrases," calling these terms "Germanisms." When we are asked to accept these locutions, he said, "we are reaching a point where agglutination resembles baby talk."

The practice of agglutinating noun (or even adjective) modifiers is anathema to translators from and into English. Other languages do not have this questionable freedom. It is painful to contemplate the conscientious translator's attempt to render (I use the word advisedly) those ponderous locutions in other languages. "Middle ear pressure" translates into French as "la pression de l'oreille moyenne"; "Eustachian tube dysfunction" as "dysfonctionnement de la trompe d'Eustache"; and "with a high bacterial level" as "à haute concentration de bactéries."

CHAPTER 15

Jargon: Medicalese, Journalese, Professionalese

Although the term *jargon* is often used pejoratively, it's not a dirty word. By definition, it is specialized language, peculiar to a category, group, or profession. Almost any group you can think of has its own inside talk, which outsiders are not expected to share.

It's one thing to use shorthand—or jargon—for convenience in conversation, in patient charts, or at medical conventions. It's quite another to use these shortcuts in serious writing.

MEDICALESE

ABNORMAL, NORMAL

X-rays are *normal* except in extraordinary circumstances. Abnormal x-rays would indeed be hazardous to one's health. What is usually meant is that the *results* or *findings* of x-ray studies or films are normal or abnormal. A more precise term is preferable for the method used, such as radiography (x-rays or gamma rays), roentgenography, or venography (phlebography).

CARDIAC DISEASE

The use of *coronary heart disease* (CHD) is medical jargon, or shorthand. The writer usually means *coronary artery disease CAD,* but since *coronary heart disease* is ambiguous, imprecise, and redundant, the attentive reader is at a loss to know just which cardiovascular disease is being referred to. Here again the temptation to use doctorese shorthand should be resisted.

Coronary artery disease refers specifically to lesions or disease of the coronary arteries and therefore should be limited to this entity.

Cardiovascular disease is often used interchangeably or synonymously with *cardiac disease*. It's true that the vascular system is almost always involved in heart disease, but there are many other cardiac aspects—electrophysiologic, chemical, electrolytic, muscular, infectious, neurologic, homeostatic, pulmonary, and congenital. The *Merck Manual* (15th ed.) described these aspects in its customary authoritative manner in a massive section titled "Cardiovascular Disorders." The term *coronary artery disease,* not *coronary heart disease,* is used throughout. There is no "coronary heart disease" entry in the manual's index.

The right coronary artery, a branch of the ascending aorta, forms an almost complete circle—crown—around the heart. So the *coronary* in *coronary artery disease* refers to the circular or coronal configuration of the *artery*, not to the heart itself.

CASES, PATIENTS, SUBJECTS, CONTROL SUBJECTS

We received three cases of essential hypertension last week.

That institution received *patients* with essential hypertension, not *cases*. A *patient* is a person who is receiving medical care.

A *case* is an instance of a disorder or disease.

A *subject* (in research or a medical investigation) is a human being or an animal with a particular characteristic. A *control subject* is one that does not have that particular characteristic in that investigation. In some investigations there may be human control subjects who are not patients, so that the use of *control patient* in that context is inaccurate.

CRITICAL

"Post Office Worker Critical after Accident." The worker's status was critical, not the worker—who was undoubtedly in no condition to complain about the medical care.

DELIVER

A woman is *delivered of* a baby. A woman gives birth. It's the physician or the midwife who *delivers* the baby, not the woman.

It might help to remember the etymology of *deliver:* from Old French *delivrer,* from Latin *de-* + *liberare,* to free, liberate.

DIAGNOSIS

It is incorrect to say "the patient was diagnosed with AIDS." Conditions, disorders, and diseases are diagnosed, not patients.

> The speech pathologist diagnosed the student's problem as one of physiologic origin.
> Economists and sociologists can diagnose the ills of a nation equally well.

DRAMATICALLY

> The incorporation of excess membrane cholesterol into an ordinarily fluid membrane can dramatically affect the physical state of the bilayer lipid.

I doubt it. High drama in the laboratory, for heaven's sake? In reality, such a setting rarely generates drama. *Dramatically* should be reserved for the theater, politics, or other histrionic pursuits.

Use instead *substantially, considerably, drastically, inordinately, extremely, severely, unduly,* or other undramatic but equally powerful and precise forms. Even *markedly*, that rather meaningless adverb so dear to the hearts of medical writers, would be preferable to *dramatically*. Such drastic changes or levels are measurable, so why not just give the relevant numbers or measurements, without the gratuitous "color"?

FALSE VERBS FROM NOUNS

> Whether the patient should be prophylaxed prior to operation remains controversial.

Antibiotics may be administered as *prophylaxis* before operations, but patients cannot possibly be prophylaxed. Nor can they be necropsied, biopsied, autopsied, or diuresed. These spuriously coined verbs, back formations, come illegitimately from legitimate nouns—*necropsy, biopsy, autopsy, diuresis.* Don't even consider using them.

Legitimate back formations include *diagnose, evaluate,* and *edit.*

Consult your dictionary if you're in doubt about which words are acceptable.

FANCY -OLOGIES

Editors groan when they see words such as *methodology* and *symptomatology.* Although these sesquipedalian words may sound authoritative, they are rarely used accurately.

Methodology is the *study* of methods, not the methods or techniques themselves. *Symptomatology* is the *study* of symptoms, not the symptoms themselves. *Etiology* is the *study* of causes, not the causes themselves, although this word may be used to indicate that *all* the causes of a particular disorder or condition are being studied, even those not immediately apparent.

> The etiology of cancer—in all its manifestations—is still mysterious.

INJECTION

Medications, preparations, and drugs are injected, not patients.

LIGATION

> I would never use a long word . . . where a short one would answer the purpose. I know there are professors in this country who "ligate" arteries. Other surgeons only tie them, and it stops the bleeding just as well.

The writer of that excerpt is Oliver Wendell Holmes, Sr.; it's from his essay titled "Scholastic and Bedside Teaching" (*Medical Essays*).

No wonder Holmes père was considered one of the best physician writers in the United States. He was also one of the most versatile, writing in several genres. Included in his best-known nonmedical works are *The Autocrat of the Breakfast Table*; the novel *Elsie Venner*; the poems *Old Ironsides*, *The Chambered Nautilus*, and *The Deacon's Masterpiece, or, The Wonderful One-Hoss Shay*; the hymn *Lord of all being! throned afar*; and the biography *Ralph Waldo Emerson*.

While he was writing these works, he was also practicing medicine in Boston and was a Professor of Anatomy at Dartmouth College (1838–1840) and at Harvard University Medical School (1847–1882).

MALE AND FEMALE

"Male and female created he them" indeed. In medical writing, as in life, a precise differentiation is possible.

> This pediatric trial comprised 50 male and 50 female patients.

By definition and context, these patients were children, of unstated age. The writer of this article—presumably the researcher as well—was in a perfect position to state the actual category at the outset: newborns or neonates (birth to 1 month of age), infants (1 month to 24 months), boys and girls (2 years to 13 years); and adolescents or teenagers (13 through 17 years). *Children* is a correct designation for people up to 13 years of age.

Teenagers may be referred to as girls and boys or as young or older teenagers.

Adult human beings (people 17 or 18 years of age and older) are referred to as *women* and *men*, not female and male, unless the cohort or study population consists of subjects of both sexes and the subjects are of unknown or indeterminable age.

MODALITY

This word is not synonymous or interchangeable with *method* or *mode*. In medicine *modality* means the method of application or use of a therapeutic agent or technique, usually a physical agent, including but not limited to massage, hydrotherapy, diathermy, or high-frequency currents.

MULTIFACTORIAL

See "Multifactorial, Multifactoral" in Chapter 12, "Dangerous Dyads and Troublesome Triads."

NOUNS AS VERBS

The English language is famous for its flexibility. Some nouns can be used as verbs, but not in these substandard sentences:

> This ruling by the legislature will impact [affect] health care [adversely?] in this state.
> You can access [reach?] [get into?] the Intensive Care Unit by that door.

ORTHODONTICS

Orthodontics is the correct word for this specialty in dentistry, which deals with correction of dentofacial abnormalities. *Orthodontia* is a synonym. "Orthodentistry" and "orthodontistry" are facetious, bogus coinages.

PARAMETER

This highly specialized word has a particular mathematical or statistical meaning, none of them a limit or boundary or (shudder) perimeter.

> The chair outlined the parameters of our responsibility.

The chair undoubtedly described the limits or the boundaries of their responsibility.

Since a *parameter* can be an independent variable *or* an arbitrary constant, as well as several other things, this word should be used cautiously. Lentner, in *Elementary Applied Statistics*, wrote that a *parameter* is a numerical quantity that might vary from one discussion to the next but is constant throughout any one discussion.

For statistics buffs, here are two other definitions (also from Lentner):

A *constant* is a numerical quantity that remains the same in every discussion.

A *variable* is a numerical quantity that might vary even throughout a single discussion.

The following sentence illustrates a correct use of *parameter*:

Hemodynamic parameters were studied before and after rapid dextran infusion.

POSITIVE

In everyday terms, a *positive* finding would be a happy one. In medical usage, such an observation might be ominous. The *results* of a "Pap" (Papanicolaou) smear could show abnormalities; that is, they could be *positive*.

PREDICTIONS OF SUDDEN DEATH

Clinical evidence of nonsustained ventricular tachycardia may predict patients at high risk of sustained arrhythmias and sudden death.

Personification (attributing human powers to inanimate or abstract objects) is perfectly good English; however, in this context it would be better to say that clinical evidence of nonsustained ventricular tachycardia may help to categorize patients at high risk of sustained arrhythmia and sudden death.

PRIOR TO, FOLLOWING

I have never found *prior to* superior to *before* in any context, and so I never use *prior to*.

As for *following,* I never use it to mean "after," preferring the simpler word. Naturally, there are times when *following* is a verb and the right word:

They are following a better course of therapy.

PROBABLE AND APPARENT DISORDERS

> He died of a probable heart attack while jogging.
> The patient succumbed to an apparent stroke during her hospitalization.

Nobody dies of a *probable* or *apparent* heart attack or stroke. They die of the real thing. It would be better to say "He apparently died of a heart attack"; "The patient apparently died of a stroke . . ."

> Three hours later, the subject developed a hypersensitivity reaction leading to expiration.

In other words, she died.

"Succumb," "expired," and "passed away" are false genteelisms. I wouldn't use "gone west" or "kicked the bucket" either if I were you.

I'm not even going to discuss "death outcome" or "condition incompatible with life."

QUANTIFY, QUANTITATE

Why do serious writers always use *quantify, quantification, quantitate* or *quantitation* when a simple *measure, measurement, determine,* or *determination* might do just as well?

Is it force of habit—that is, using a longer word when a simpler one would do? Is it a questionable quirk, a pedantic, polysyllabic predilection, or merely sesquipedalianism *gratia* sesquipedalianism?

SERVES AS

> He is a world-renowned internist and serves as the editor of a famous medical journal.

What's wrong with just plain "and is the editor of a famous medical journal"?

SUSPICIOUS

Pathologic, cytologic, or laboratory results are not *suspicious*. If they are uncertain, and if the clinician is unable to reach a definitive conclusion concerning the diagnosis or the gravity of the patient's condition, the results may be referred to as *inconclusive* or *questionable.* There is certainly no need to frighten the patient by using a phrase such as "suspicious findings."

TITRATION

This is an incorrect usage:

> Patients should then be titrated on the basis of antiarrhythmic response and tolerance.

Titration is the measurement or analysis of a particular component in a solution by means of a reagent; therefore, patients cannot be titrated. If jargon can be said to be pure, the sentence quoted above, from a journal article, is pure jargon.

JOURNALESE AND PROFESSIONALESE

Journalese is characterized by non sequiturs, dangling modifiers and other evidences of careless or reckless grammar, and imprecise statements.

Competent journalists pay attention to good grammar and usage. They avoid "cutesy" and slangy, overly breezy phraseology, preferring to base their reputation for professionalism on accuracy and appropriately colorful phraseology.

Medical journalists in a free society have a special obligation: to present the facts impartially after doing their homework.

The American people owe a tremendous debt of gratitude to these professionals working in the print and electronic media, who have done so much to educate the public about the danger signals of cancer, the penalties of smoking, the latest advances in medical knowledge and technology, and the practical limitations as well as the great accomplishments of physicians and other medical workers.

ARGUABLY

I had never seen this word in formal writing until fairly recently. It is often mistakenly used to mean "inarguably" ("unarguably"), that is, "without a doubt." *Arguably* means that the point can be argued, that is, it is questionable or debatable.

AUTHOR

Use of *author* as a verb meaning "to write" is pretentious and unnecessary. Plain old *wrote* is fine.

Author as a noun is also fine.

BITES AND BYTES

> Medical celebrities can use sound bytes productively for public education.

It should be "sound *bites,*" if that term must be used. A *byte* (the term was first recorded officially in 1962, probably as a variant of *bite*) is right out of computerland and is defined as a group of adjacent *b*inary digits that a computer processes as a unit.

A sound bite, which could also be called (but not by me) an "audio opportunity," is a quotable statement, usually in a political context. The term originates with the idea that a sound editor (an audio editor, that is—an unsound editor is unthinkable) cuts ("bites") a telling excerpt from a tape for future use.

BUREAUCRATESE

Back in 1981, Malcolm Baldrige, then Commerce Secretary, sick and tired of bureaucratese—language beloved of government jobholders—circulated a memorandum to all employees in his department listing 43 words and phrases he did not care to see in office correspondence.

His *index expurgatorius* included *bottom line, finalize, great majority, input, interface, maximize, prioritize, viable,* and *impact* as a verb.

I wonder how successful Baldrige was. Has anyone ever done a follow-up study?

BURGEONING

This word means budding, not mushrooming, proliferating, or growing uncontrollably.

BUST, ARREST

In serious writing or radio or television broadcasts, the term *bust* to mean arrest has become ubiquitous, not to say monotonous. Could we forgo this bit of slang? This request is addressed particularly to television broadcasters, who are looked upon by average citizens as paragons of good taste in English.

BUZZ WORDS

This nonce term reminds me of the practical joker who delivers an electrical jolt as he genially holds out his hand in greeting.

Avoid using "buzz word" and buzz words in general. They include Malcolm Baldrige's little list of words that never would be missed, *knowledgewise* and other bizarre *-wises, cohort* used incorrectly, *mickey mouse* for amateurish, *candy store* problem, *déjà vu, nostalgia,* and the ubiquitous and tiresome *bottom line* (correct, however, when used in bookkeeping or accounting).

CONTACT, COMMUNICATE

Many editors and writers consider *contact* to be jargon when it is used as a verb. The mere thought of "contacting" anyone physically (especially in hot weather) is repugnant to some people.

Because I consider the one word (in this instance) preferable to a wordy, awkward phrase such as "get in touch with," an ambiguous term such as "reach," or a stilted phrase such as "get in communication with," I do use *contact* in informal writing, but never in serious writing, in which I specify the mode of communication.

CUTTING EDGE

This phrase is used synonymously with "leading edge." Both phrases are overused. I think they mean something like the "vanguard."

DIALOGUE

Despite Shakespeare ("and dialogued for him what he would say"), I prefer to limit the use of *dialogue* to its function as a noun.

DRAMATICALLY

See this entry under "Medicalese" in this chapter.

EARLY ON

Researchers determined early on that cholinergic neurons are destroyed in patients with senile dementia.

For some reason obscure to me (but perhaps because it sounds so, so British), this phrase has become voguish. *Early* is good enough.

FOR FREE

Each registrant was given a parcel of goodies for free.

Free; the "for" is annoying and always redundant.

FREE GIFT

No serious writer would willingly use this term. However, marketing researchers tell me that the public responds more strongly to the word *free* in advertisements than to any other word.

Given this piece of intelligence, one can better understand the seeming redundancy. *Gift* falls pleasantly enough on the ear, and *free* rings a bell.

GOT TO BE

There's got to be a better way to diagnose Alzheimer's disease.

Popularizing medical works is the best way to educate the public. However, that sentence is too breezy, even for the medical center's newsletter in which it appeared. The elision in this instance is substandard—it stands for "there has got to be," an awkward if not downright ungrammatical locution. In other words, it would be fine in conversation but not in a medical newsletter.

In serious writing there is a fine line between an informal style and "we're all just folks here." It takes a gift for the language or fine craftsmanship to discern the line and observe it:

There must be a better way to diagnose Alzheimer's disease.

HEAD UP

The board chose an expert on infectious diseases to head up the hospital utilization committee.

To head is sufficient.

JARGONWISE

Grafting *-wise* onto more than one word in any one piece, especially when it is an unknown coinage, brands the perpetrator as a lazy writer. Either that or the purported author doesn't own a thesaurus.

This suffix—serviceable when used sparingly and wisely—is from Old English *wisan*, meaning manner.

A word to the wise: one *-wise* to an article.

THE LAZARUS SYNDROME

Anachronistic references to the *late* so-and-so (and often she or he was a so-and-so) are usually redundant. It is unnecessary to say, for instance, "He was considerably indebted to the late Sir William Osler," since "the late" designations should generally be confined to those who have died recently, say within the last 5 or 10 years. Well-known, notorious, or celebrated persons or personages need not be so designated, since it is assumed that *everyone* knows who they were and also knows they are dead.

Such ex post facto (after-the-fact) formulations can lead to absurdities and redundancies such as "the widower married the late Prudence Cash in Canada." She was not dead at the time of the wedding.

> The late Juliet Stratford, grandmother of the groom, completed the wedding party.

A macabre thought.

> The deceased was offered the option of a second medical opinion.

Too late.

The handy phrase *ex post facto* can be used as either an adjective or an adverb: "ex post facto judgments" ("Monday morning quarterback"); "accusations of misfeasance were made ex post facto."

The antonym of *ex post* is *ex ante*.

PALPABLE

To say that the "excitement was palpable" is not only a cliche but pure hyperbole. Ask any cardiologist or gastroenterologist.

A rapid pulse or an enlarged liver or spleen can be *palpable*, that is, capable of being touched or felt. The excitement could be *nearly* palpable.

PERSONNEL

This impersonal word can usually be replaced by *employees* when individuals are meant. It refers to a body or group of persons in a particular organization or firm.

Sometimes it is necessary to use *personnel*, as in military personnel and personnel administration or management (which encompasses the entire body of employees as well as single [or married] employees).

PLUS

This all-purpose word is often used incorrectly:

> Use of the laser in this setting is efficient, plus it's advantageous to the rest of the operating room team.

Plus can be a noun, an adjective, a verb, or a preposition, but never a conjunction. It is correctly used to mean "in addition to":

> Psychiatrists prescribe an antidepressant plus supplemental hormonal therapy for this disorder.

SAVING AND SAVINGS

The plural *savings* is correctly used in the following sentences:

> They lost their entire savings during the Depression.
> A savings account is a sound financial cushion.

A current solecism is the use of the plural *savings* when the singular *saving* is correct: "a saving of $50." This usage is particularly pervasive in retail merchandising. Let us hope that in time this currency will cease to be minted.

SKILL AND SKILLS

Only *skill* is needed—as in reading skill, verbal skill, writing skill.

Adding an *s* to *skill* in these terms is painting the lily or gilding refined gold. In other words, the *s* is redundant:

> Poor writing skills are the most common weakness of young executives.

> Poor writing skill certainly is the most common weakness.

SUFFRAGETTE, SUFFRAGIST

The proper term for a proponent of votes for women is *suffragist*, whether woman or man. *Suffragette* is, like *usherette, poetess, coed* (to mean only women students), and *authoress,* insufferably supercilious.

TITULAR PUNCTUATION

Don't use a comma if the title precedes the name.

> Former National Institutes of Health Director, James B. Wyngaarden, is an eminent physician.

The commas should be deleted. The sentence then becomes nonjargonistic, journalistically speaking.

The sentence could also have read: "The former Director of the National Institutes of Health, James B. Wyngaarden, . . ."

"TYPES"

> Environmental types quickly came on the scene to evaluate the damage to beaches.

The writer should have written "environmental experts," "representatives of the Environmental Protection Agency," if that is what is meant, or, if they are protesters, "environmental activists."

"Types" is just a "tad" (don't use this obnoxious word in formal writing either) too imprecise to be used by people who purport to be professional journalists.

UNDERCAPITALIZED

> If it had not been for the state's catastrophic insurance director, the Health Department would never have learned of this disaster.

A small disaster, journalistically speaking, easily remedied by capitalizing in the proper places.

Such gaffes could be obviated by bending the journalistic rule that titles are not capitalized unless they precede the name of the titleholder.

Just a suggestion: The reporter (or rewrite person) could write something like "The Catastrophic Insurance Director, Penelope Diamantis, saved the day by . . ." or could be creative and use a hyphen: "Catastrophic-Insurance Director . . ."

ADVICE

Don't use bad jargon.
Save the good jargon for conversation.

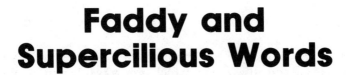

CHAPTER 16

Faddy and Supercilious Words

Certain words and catchphrases come into vogue, have their brief day in the sun, and mercifully vanish. Who is there now to mourn "Try it, you'll like it"?

Some terms should not be used at all in serious writing, and some should not be used except correctly and in a noncondescending way.

ARMAMENTARIUM

I have never felt the need to use *armamentarium*. Try instead available resources, equipment, methods, information, collection, or array, in accordance with your meaning.

FANTASTIC

Theoretically almost anything goes in conversation. We can therefore excuse "fantastic!" as a vulgate expression of enthusiasm—if it is used only once per customer per conversation. Hearing this word over and over again is wearisome. It ranks (and I mean that) with "terrific!" and the infuriating "you know" used as punctuation in every sentence.

In writing, the designation *fantastic* should be confined to fictional dialogue, Tinkerbell, the Wizard of Oz, the minotaur, centaurs, satyrs, nymphs, mythology, and other such fantastical fabrications.

LIAISE

This spurious back formation (from *liaison*, a legitimate noun, taken bodily from French) deserves a speedy demise.

Liaison (pronounced lee-ay-zon or lee-ə-zon, but not lay-ə-zon) is from the French *lier*, to tie or bind, plus *-aison*, the French version of the English *-ation* and the Latin *-ation-* or *-atio*.

LIVID

Despite popular belief, one who becomes *livid* with rage does not turn purple—he or she becomes ashen pale. *Livid* comes from the Latin *lividus*, meaning lead-colored.

MAJOR

One of the most abused, overused, and misused words of this generation is the adjective *major*, which is mistakenly written or spoken to connote the most important or significant.

Major, exactly the same in English and Latin, is the comparative of the Latin *magnus*, meaning large or great. *Major*, being merely a comparative, therefore means larg*er* or great*er*, not great*est* or larg*est*. The superlative of *magnus* is *maximus*.

A few alternatives to *major*—depending on the meaning—besides *greater* are *important, chief, main, superior, larger, serious, considerable, impressive,* and *principal.*

NEEDLESS TO SAY

Needless to say is not only supercilious—it is redundant. If something is needless to say, why say it?

OBVIOUSLY, CLEAR

Obviously implies all that is supercilious and condescending in writing. Another such word is *clear.* The very word *supercilious* comes from the Latin word for eyebrow, *supercilium,* from *super,* above, and *cilium,* the eyelid.

These words can be used appropriately, that is, without patronizing the reader:

The patient was obviously suffering respiratory distress.

In this instance, *obviously* is used to mean that the patient's distress was plain for all to see; there is no condescension here.

Their investigation and results were obviously flawed.

To whom was the flaw obvious? The writer is saying in effect that any fool could plainly see what was wrong. If so, one is constrained to comment that the granting agency didn't get its money's worth from this investigation.

It was clear that more than one factor was responsible for this finding.

Again—to whom was it clear? The writer should state the conclusion or thought without the nonattributable opening phrase.

See also "Superciliousness and Condescension" in Chapter 13, "Tautology."

PREVENTATIVE

If you remember *prevent*, you'll never use the obsolete "preventative" instead of *preventive*. The noun is *prevention*, not "preventation."

SCENARIO

This word should be restricted to the making of films and the movies. If one feels impelled to use it otherwise, one should not use it more than once a month.

STATE OF THE ART

If this phrase comes after the verb in a sentence, don't hyphenate it:

Their management and treatment of cancer were state of the art.

If *state of the art* is used at all (and I wish it weren't overused), it should be hyphenated when it becomes a compound adjective preceding the noun it modifies:

That state-of-the-art piece of technology, the computer, had created a revolution in information storage, retrieval, and documentation.

VIABLE

In former times, one never saw the word *viable* except in a medical sense, meaning something that is capable of existing independently, on its own—a fetus, for example. Today it is used incorrectly to mean feasible, workable, "doable," practical, practicable, and possible.

Carried to its illogical conclusion, this word is a travesty:

They came to believe that suicide was the only viable alternative to a lingering death.

Should we writers and editors laugh or cry?
Let us preserve the nice, precise meaning of *viable*.

CHAPTER 17

English as She Is Spoke

American English is a strange and wondrous language.

The student asks, "How come 'fat chance' and 'slim chance' mean the same thing?" Or "slow up" and "slow down"?

How is it that Oscar Wilde's epigram, "I can resist everything but temptation," can be misquoted as "I can resist anything but temptation" and still mean the same?

The answer is, "It's idiomatic. Idioms are special ways to say certain things. There is no logic to many of our Americanisms. That's just the way it is."

Other languages are no different. Remember the *gallicismes* you learned in high school? *Comment allez-vous?* How do you go? This French question translates freely as "How are you?" *Faire ses choux gras* literally means to make one's cabbages fat; in everyday language it means to feather one's nest.

In Yiddish, to *hock a cheynick* literally means to bang a teakettle, but the intended meaning is to nag or to engage in irritating and provocative repetition—something *noodges* engage in. Transliteration and phonetic spelling are always controversial, so you may—and might—spell those terms differently.

Follett says: "Any locution, especially when long established, is entitled to a reasonable interpretation of its intent. A self-addressed envelope is not one that addressed itself: it is an envelope addressed to oneself."

HOW'S THAT AGAIN?

Involuntary overhearers who write for a living use everything as grist, including conversations in buses or restaurants. Here are some malapropisms, tidbits, or utterances, heard or seen—just a letter, a word, or a sound off the real thing:

When he referred to Genesis 47:28, he quoted Ver Batem.

Luckily they had ballet parking at the airport.

Every ambassador then in Washington was invited to a steak dinner at the White House.

High rollers go to Atlantic City to play Bacharach.

The plaintiff thought he could get off with a flea bargain.

Barcelona was fascinating—we saw flamingo dancers.

I don't think you can blanketly say that drug dealers shouldn't be used as witnesses.

The agitated patient wrestled [wrested] the vial away from the physician.

Parishioners there pray to Our Lady of Perpetual Health. [Perhaps the patron saint of physicians.]

Never leave off tomorrow what you can do today.

The assailant explained that he had been "thoroughly provocated."

I don't have to take any of your gruff.

They ran the whole gambit from A to Z.

The chapel has a caustic ceiling.

Her grant proposal was put together in a slaphazard way.

The deceased was funeralized on Friday and interned at Mount Joseph Cemetery.

Verbatim quotation from an interview with a preacher:

Fornification is a sin.

The columnist Jeff Greenfield wrote that a broadcaster on a New York television station actually said this:

Today the Pope beautified a caramelized nun.

OTHER VULGATE EXPRESSIONS

AS FAR AS

Many people never go as far as they should.

As far as the welfare of the nurses, I believe it is at stake.
They went as far as the corner store.

The second cited sentence is correct. The first should have read, "As far as the welfare of the nurses *is concerned*, I believe it is at stake."

BASICALLY

One thorn in the flesh of good editors is the thoughtless use of *basically*, especially at the beginning of a sentence. It rarely means *fundamentally.* Often it is used as a transition word or to gain time in speech. What is usually meant is *mainly, principally, chiefly,* or *actually.*

Basically may be supplanting *hopefully* as the most obnoxious dangler or, like, you know, punctuation.

In serious writing, *basically* should not be used at the head of a sentence; if it is used within a sentence, it should mean *fundamentally* or *essentially.* It's another of those catch-all words that poor conversationalists find so handy.

> The solution was basically neutral.

The previous sentence, from a junior high school laboratory report, is basically a pun but a chemist would find fault with it.

BETTER

> They better look at the electrocardiogram one more time.

Grammatically and medically speaking, they *had better* look at the ECG once again.

CONSIDERS OR CONSIDERS AS

> The entire region considers him as one of the finest teachers in Illinois.

There is a subtlety involved in whether to use *as* in certain sentences. The sentence could have two meanings: If *as* is used, it means that the region is giving him consideration as a fine teacher, perhaps with a view to appointing him state secretary of education. If *as* is deleted, it means that the region is of the opinion that he is a fine teacher.

COUP DE GRACE

The correct phrase, from the French, is *coup de grace* (not "coup de gras"), the "death blow of mercy," to end the misery of an animal or a human being.

Coup means blow or stroke; *gras* means fat. Therefore, a *coup de gras* would be a stroke of fat—not a pretty picture.

This French phrase has been integrated into the English language, and so any accent is unnecessary. However, if you wish, you may include the circumflex accent over the *a* in *grâce.*

COUPLE

The philanthropist left a couple million dollars to the Cystic Fibrosis Foundation.

A fine and laudable bequest, but the expression is slangy. He left a couple *of* million dollars.

If you mean two, say *two*—rather than *couple of.*

FACILITY

The use of *facility* to mean a concrete (I use the word wittingly) structure is substandard. It is far better to use a word describing the actual edifice: clinic, building, wing, department, suite, medical center, hospital, emergency room, laboratory, operating room.

HOPEFULLY

Hopefully means "with hope" or "in a hopeful manner." Any other use is laying an undue burden on this potentially valuable word.

> The institute's findings will hopefully lay the groundwork for the future as the legislature begins to consider and hopefully act on these recommendations.

Too many *hopefully*s in that actual magazine clipping. The trouble with this monotonous and repugnant word (only when it's used incorrectly) is that no one reading the sentence knows who is doing the hoping.

This convoluted sentence would better have read, "We hope the institute's findings will lay the groundwork as the legislature considers and acts on these recommendations."

If *hopefully* stands at the head of a sentence, you can almost always be sure that it is being used with the implicit meaning of "I [or we] hope." However, is that what is meant in the following sentence?

> Hopefully they returned to the therapist.

They returned to the therapist with hope? Or we hope they returned to the therapist?

> Hopefully the nephrologists can treat incontinence medically rather than surgically.

We hope that they can do so? Or do the nephrologists hope?

If it is not already an L.C., we writers and editors would do well to campaign for eradication of its incorrect use.

I write this essay hopefully.

THE MEANHIM (HIMANME) SYNDROME

> Me and him had to go to the emergency room.

A long time ago, teachers taught that *I* (the speaker) always came last in a series of two or more. I concur with that (outdated?) grammar and philosophy. *Me* and *him* are the objective, not the nominative, case.

> He and I had to go to the emergency room.

I've been amazed to hear *me* and *him* used as nominatives by presumably educated (informed) people. Many professional athletes also seem to suffer from this syndrome (even former collegians), perhaps because it is difficult to express oneself in the shower room when a "mike" is thrust in one's face, or perhaps because they feel impelled to maintain their machismo or a rugged image. However, bad grammar is neither a validation nor a sine qua non of athleticism.

MORE IMPORTANT(LY)

If one regards *more important* or *more importantly* as transitional phrases used to begin the next sentence with, there may be reason to use one or the other.

If *more important* means "what is more important," then this adjective is correct. The difficulty with this reasoning is that the word after the bridging phrase may be a noun, in which case the phrase may be misread as modifying that noun.

It is probable that *more importantly* would be correct in all instances. Although it is not a participial phrase, it is considered an absolute construction—a phrase that is grammatically unconnected with the rest of the sentence. (Most absolute constructions are participial phrases.)

> More important, the patient with hepatitis was returned to the intensive care unit.

Does that mean that this particular patient was more important than, say, one with congestive heart failure? If the bridging phrase modifies the entire sentence (the more common use), the "sentence adverb" *more importantly* is correct.

> More importantly, triage was performed within minutes after the derailment.

I have never used either expression.

NOT LIKE YOU LIKE IT

> A Chicago-area educator has been ordered to pay his ex-wife half his take-home pay for the next four years so that she, like he, can attain a doctoral degree.

Let us hope that the writer of this article can attain some semblance of good grammar, without a doctoral degree. Make it "so that she, like *him* . . ."

Like as a preposition takes the objective case.

The grammatically insecure are so afraid of using *like* incorrectly that they use *like they are* instead of plain *like them*.

Despite Winston, which "tastes good like a cigarette should," *like* is *never* a conjunction. This ungrammatical cigarette advertisement—which apparently had a larger audience than did the still, small voice muttering that *like* is not a conjunction—is undoubtedly responsible for the unshakable belief of an entire generation that *like* is a conjunction. One can only hope that this false dictum is set not in granite but in smoke rings.

A quick test will tell you whether you should use *like*: If *as if* will do, *like* is incorrect.

Like can also be an adjective (they possess *like* attributes) and a noun (*like* calls to *like*).

Sometimes the writer is so nervous about making an error in using *like* that a worse error is made:

> We hope that this edition, as its predecessor editions, will be a valuable source of information.

Like its predecessor editions. *As* is incorrect. Besides, as Theodore Bernstein wrote (*Watch Your Language*), it sounds as hell.

PODIUM

> Many lecturers find it difficult to stand almost motionless behind the podium; they prefer to walk back and forth.

Make that "behind the lectern."

This word is often misused instead of *lectern*.

The *podium* is the raised platform on which you stand or the dais at which you sit. When you rise to speak, you stand behind the lectern, a reading desk, which is usually furnished with a lamp.

Podium is taken bodily from the Latin, but in Latin it means a balcony or, by extension, a raised area. The plural is *podiums* or *podia*.

PREPOSITIONS AND OBJECTIVE CASE

> This matter is strictly between he and I.

The correct version:

> This matter is strictly between him and me.

Between is a preposition, and the noun or pronoun in the phrase is its object. In English, nouns are not inflected, so that their nominative and objective cases are the same. However, this is not the case with pronouns.

> This is a great honor for my colleague and I.

Wrong. My colleague and *me*.

> Dr. Butler's loss will be deeply felt by we in Ohio who relied on his wisdom.

By *us*, whether in Ohio or elsewhere.

PROHIBITION IS FORBIDDEN

To forbid is often used interchangeably and mistakenly for *to prohibit.*

Although the two verbs are virtually synonymous, *forbid* should be followed by *to* and *prohibit* by *from*. "Prohibit to" and "forbid from" are always incorrect. These sentences are correct:

> The attending physician's policy is to forbid patients with Buerger's disease to smoke.
> Visitors are prohibited from smoking in rooms containing oxygen tanks or tents.

If a mnemonic association is needed, try Bernstein's: "4bid 2." Unfortunately, *prohibit* doesn't lend itself to this kind of numerate aid.

REFLEXIVES

It's not good practice to use "what sounds good" when deciding whether to use *me* or *myself.* The same goes for all the other *-self* words, known in the grammar trade as reflexives.

The rules are simple: The "-self" or "-selves" words are used for two purposes: first, to emphasize ("Mother, I'd rather do it myself"), and second, reflexively, so that the action is turned back on the grammatical subject:

> I never quite accustomed myself to the altitude of Denver.
> The dermatologist learned that the patients had overexposed themselves to ultraviolet radiation from tanning devices.

The stilted use of reflexive pronouns indicates the grammatical insecurity of the writer or speaker. Plain old *me* (or any other plain old unreflexive pronoun) is correct.

> There is no question of harmony between him and myself.

Since there is no reflexive action, it should read "between him and *me*."

THOSE KIND

> Those kind of things—delayed blood chemistry results—make any clinician impatient.

There is no correct phrase such as "those kind," only *that kind* or *those kinds. That* and *kind* are singulars and *those* and *kinds* are plural. They should not be intermixed.

One hears the illiterate, incongruous "those kind" too often from people who should know better.

UNIQUE PRONUNCIATION

Although *u* is ordinarily a vowel, it can have the sound of *y*, a consonant. Use *a*, not *an*:

> *a* unique diagnostic tool
> *a* ubiquitous presence
> *a* unanimous decision
> *a* UCLA student
> *a* U.S.P. formulary

VERBALLY AND ORALLY

The distinction between these words is important. *Verbal* has to do with words generally, and *oral* has to do with the spoken word, so that the proper use of *oral* is more circumscribed.

> Two members of the house staff received letters of reprimand, and the third was criticized verbally.

Most criticism is accomplished with words, although eyebrows or other body parts may be raised for the same purpose. (The raised finger comes to mind.) In the example, the writer probably meant that the third member was given a tongue-lashing—a literally *oral* criticism.

See also "Verbal, oral" in Chapter 12, "Dangerous Dyads and Troublesome Triads."

WHENCE

He was transferred to a medical center in the Midwest, the region from whence he had come some years ago.

Whence means "from where," and so "from whence" is redundant. The sentence should read, "the region whence he had come" if the writer feels the need to use this obsolescent word.

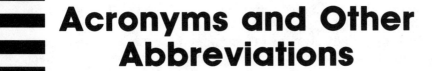

CHAPTER 18

Acronyms and Other Abbreviations

Acronyms, initialisms (initializations), symbols, or shortened forms—all are abbreviations: WASP, acronym; IHSS, initialism; mg, sec, U, p.o., b.i.d., abbreviations or shortened forms. Abbreviations include symbols as well: $, &, %.

ACRONYMS AND INITIALISMS

Acronyms are formed from the initial letters of a term or parts of a term.

Just any old initialism or abbreviation consisting of all capitals cannot be termed an acronym. Acronyms are upper crust. To make the grade as an acronym, the item, whether or not all caps, must be capable of being pronounced as a word.

The expressions OED, FDA, FACP, MRI, NDA, NSAID, FBI, CBS, PT, NYU, XL, and SGPT are not acronyms—they're initialisms. The expressions CAD, AIDS, laser, DESI, sonar, snafu, scuba, MeSH, ZIP, COBOL, and SADS are acronyms. The computer-generated indexing system of the National Library of Medicine, MEDLARS is an acronym, as are POMP and SCRAP. LED is the acronym for light-emitting diode.

Sonar was formerly known as ASDIC, for Antisubmarine Detection Investigation Committee, a group formed during World War I that engendered manufacture of the device. The term *sonar* (sound navigation and ranging) came into use in World War II.

USING ABBREVIATIONS

In medical manuscripts it is judicious and customary to spell out a long or complicated term the first time it is used in the text, with the shortened form given in parentheses immediately following. Thereafter in the manuscript, the shortened form may be used if it is an accepted, common abbreviation.

Government agencies and certain organizations or groups often use initials for their names. Good practice mandates full spelling of the name at first mention, even if "everybody in the country knows what *FDA* stands for"; the name may then be abbreviated throughout the work.

If a term is used only two or three times throughout the work, don't abbreviate it. If the work is long and several pages intervene between mentions, spell out the term again, to remind the reader what the abbreviation stands for.

Avoid starting a sentence (footnotes are exceptions) with a number or an abbreviation, especially a Greek letter or other such symbol.

Good writers and editors never forget that scholars and others throughout the world read American publications. No reader in Kenya or Tierra del Fuego should be frustrated by encountering a mysterious abbreviation. In America "No" means "no," but in France or Italy it can stand for *numero*, "number."

One of the greatest vexations for readers of medical works is the peppering of initialisms and other abbreviations throughout an article or book. This overdose sometimes means that the unfortunate reader must turn back several pages to discover what the author meant by that obscure abbreviation. After several interruptions, the reader loses interest and thus misses the point of the article and the reason for its existence as well.

Jawbreakers such as *idiopathic hypertrophic subaortic stenosis* (IHSS) are understandably always abbreviated throughout a work after first mention. Indeed, some journals state in their instructions to authors that abbreviations such as DNA, EDTA, pH, RNA, UHF, and VHF need not be spelled out at all, since these terms are universally understood and are unambiguous.

Don't initial-cap spelled-out terms that are then abbreviated all-caps:

> The new team is conducting research on temporomandibular joint (TMJ) disorders [not Temporomandibular Joint Disorders].
>
> The diagnosis was made after magnetic resonance imaging [not Magnetic Resonance Imaging] (MRI).

Greek letters, P or *P* for probability (follow house style), S.E.M. (or SEM, standard error of the mean), S.D. (or SD, standard deviation of a sample), the symbols for greater than ($>$) and less than ($<$), and other such symbols need not be spelled out. The writer certainly may choose to spell out the abbreviation anyway in a footnote or in parentheses within the text.

If the manuscript looks as if it suffers from alphabet soup syndrome, delete all but two or three universal, traditional abbreviations and continue to spell out the rest, no matter how tiresome it may seem to you. Brevity can spell CATASTROPHE. (I'm waiting for some organization to come up with this one. If it already exists, please let me know.) Economy is good, but not at the expense of clarity. As Horace wrote in *Ars Poetica*, "*Brevis esse laboro, obscurus fio*" ("In laboring to be brief, I become obscure").

Many medical journals frown on ad hoc abbreviations and do not permit their authors to use them at all. Being scholarly, their editors know it would be impossible for all readers to be conversant with the terminologies of all disciplines.

This prohibition against author-coined abbreviations is understandable: They mean different things to different people. The dangers inherent in *initialese* are evident when one discovers that PT stands for at least 30 entities, including the following, depending on the specialty or subspecialty: physical therapy, physical therapist, patient, point, part, posterior tibial (artery), prothrombin time, pint, perstetur (let it be continued), parathyroid, paroxysmal tachycardia, permanent and total, pneumothorax, and pharmacology and therapeutics.

The same goes for O.D.: To the ophthalmologist, optician, or optometrist, O.D. means the right eye (oculus dexter), but it also stands for Doctor of Optometry, officer of the day, every day (omni die), overdose, optimal dose, outside diameter, and doubtlessly many other things as well.

To the nurse and the patient, TLC means tender, loving care. To the researcher it may mean thin-layer chromatography; to the pulmonary specialist, total lung capacity.

GU can mean gastric ulcer to a gastroenterologist, genitourinary to a urologist, or glycogenic unit to other kinds of specialists.

TV can mean television, tidal volume, total volume, tetrazolium violet, trial visit, *Trichomonas vaginalis*, trichomoniasis vaginitis, or tuberculin volutin, not to mention thoracic vertebrae, tickborne virus, toxic vertigo, transvenous, trivalent, tricuspid valve, truncal vagotomy, or typhus vaccine.

To politics buffs, Mao was the Chairman, but in medicine MAO means monoamine oxidase (MAOI is its inhibitor), maximal acid output, and Master of the Art of Obstetrics.

The exotic QUICHA may look like a South American language to some, a variation of a tasty dish to others. However, to pulmonologists it means quantitative inhalation challenge apparatus.

Computerized (axial) tomography was formerly abbreviated CAT, but is now just CT for even more brevity. Child's apperception test, chronic abdominal tympany, and computer of average transients are abbreviated CAT.

To a pulmonologist, SOB means dyspnea—shortness of breath. However, there are other meanings in other disciplines.

It was probably inattention that caused this infelicitous absurdity from a case report:

> A 15-year-old patient with diabetes and a skin ulcer developed a deterioration of renal and liver function with a rising bun.

One can only speculate what else might have resulted in a rising BUN.

MEDLARS, MEDLINE, MeSH

The acronym MEDLARS, the registered initialism for Medical Literature Analysis and Retrieval System, stands for the medical literature retrieval services of the National Library of Medicine, which publishes our old and dear friend *Index Medicus.*

The acronym MEDLINE comes from MEDLARS "on line."

The acronym MeSH stands for medical subject headings used by the National Library of Medicine in indexing and cataloging materials.

MNEMONIC AIDS

Acronymy is widespread and fashionable because it provides a built-in mnemonic association. This is an advantage in our society, so impatient and so receptive to public relations urgings. Organizations have been known to create acronyms and then coin their ad hoc names to fit the acronyms. It works—people tend to remember acronyms more readily than lengthy expressions.

The acronym NOW is easier to remember than National Organization for Women, and one doesn't have to worry about whether it's "of" or "for" women.

I too have been guilty of coining mnemonic aids, for myself and for my students. CAPERS, for example, represents all that is necessary in medical writing:

> *c*larity
> *a*ccuracy
> *p*reciseness
> *e*conomy
> *r*eflectiveness
> *s*implicity

Another acronym I've coined is NAILS, which embodies all that should be avoided in medical writing:

> *n*onsense
> *a*mbiguity

*i*llogic
*l*ogodaedaly
*s*loth

As defined in *Webster III*, *logodaedaly* is the arbitrary or capricious coinage of words.

Acronyms and other abbreviations are especially handy and popular in conversation. If the abbreviation or acronym starts with the sound of a vowel, use *an*; if with the sound of a consonant, use *a*:

an NIH grant
a B.S. degree in library science
an NYU graduate
an 1130

Even in the same medical institution, it may be impossible to standardize terms, and certainly an abbreviated term should never be used to mean two different things in the same specialty or subspecialty.

Physicians should use "COPD" (chronic obstructive pulmonary disease) rather than "COLD" on the patient's chart, for fear of having a serious disorder misread as just a garden-variety upper respiratory infection.

A frustrated attending physician sometimes enters GOK on a patient's chart; it means "God only knows."

As far as I know, ZIP as in "code" has no meaning other than the original one, Zone Improvement Plan (or Program); "zip" conveys the idea of speed. It was a brilliant concept, and it has succeeded. This expression is always written all-caps.

PERIODS IN ABBREVIATIONS

Acronyms should not have periods within them and are not ordinarily followed by periods except at the end of a sentence.

Some publishers of books and journals do not use periods in such abbreviations as M.D. and Pharm. D. and thus write them solid: MD, PharmD. Follow the prescribed house style of the publisher or journal.

Periods are ordinarily used in pharmacy terms such as b.i.d., t.i.d., and p.o. to avoid even the faintest possibility of misunderstanding a prescription or a patient's chart.

PLURALS OF ABBREVIATIONS

There is no need to add an apostrophe to pluralize all-caps acronyms or other initialisms: ECGs (note that EKG should not be used in English); CVAs; WASPs.

Since the plural is implicit, an *s* is not necessary to pluralize lowercase abbreviations that do not have internal or terminal periods: mg, cm, mL. However, abbreviations that have internal periods are pluralized with an apostrophe and *s*: r.b.c.'s; w.b.c.'s. (*RBC*s and *WBC*s are also correct.)

GLOSSARY

In a lengthy work encompassing many necessary initialisms or other abbreviations, the medical writer might well consider appending a glossary of these terms for the reader's convenience and quick reference.

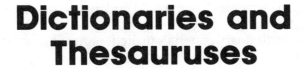

Dictionaries and Thesauruses

In citing the *Random House Dictionary of the English Language,* 2d ed., 1987, William Safire, who writes a delightful feature column on politics and English usage in the *New York Times,* recommends that the dictionary "should report the language as used, and it should also specify when usage is considered slang or substandard."

The question is, "as used by whom?" Some words and phrases spoken or written by the average citizen may be appropriate in conversation. Certain radio or television offerings, with their pseudo-folksy utterances, are carefully prepared to appeal to those the network executives consider to be at a fourth-grade comprehension level.

Writing—particularly formal and expository writing—is far different from conversation. Color and imagery are desirable in that kind of writing too, but not at the expense of preciseness, accuracy, good taste, and clarity.

Instituting an Académie Américaine to parallel the Académie Française would be absurd in light of our justly famous freedom of usage; to say that there should be no standards would be equally absurd. As usual, the sensible, reasonable answer is somewhere in the middle. But my middle is weighted on the side of the excellent writers and speakers in this country, not the speechifiers or the poorly educated or prepared, anything-goes population.

A recent edition of the Académie Française dictionary has added almost a thousand new borrowings, based mainly on English scientific and technical words and phrases. These additions are *"babélismes,"* defined in the new edition as the "degradation of a language by the invasion of foreign words."

Most endeavors—whether dentistry, the law, genetics, engineering and technology of all kinds, biology, horticulture, music, library science, and certainly medicine, nursing, and pharmaceuticals—require preciseness in language so that students and readers of these bodies of literature can comprehend readily.

DICTIONARIES AND THESAURUSES **169**

The makers of dictionaries are continuously engaged in searching for new words and usages. They consider dictionaries not arbiters of style but records of a living language.

The publisher's preface to the 24th edition of *Stedman's* puts it sagaciously: "Like any dictionary, *Stedman's* is a tool and, as with any newly acquired instrument, one should understand the directions for its use before attempting to use it."

Look on preliminary materials in dictionaries as users' manuals.

DICTIONARIES FOR BAD SPELLERS

Poor spellers are happy to know that there are dictionaries written especially for them. These books can be found in the reference section of many book stores.

See Chapter 10, "Commonly Misspelled Words," for more on this kind of dictionary.

THESAURUSES

The sheer scholarliness of these treasures (the literal meaning of *thesaurus* is storehouse or treasure chamber) is staggering. My library contains a goodly number of them; they have often saved my sanity and my valuable time.

It should be remembered that thesauruses are not dictionaries— that is, they don't define words. They merely give the user ideas as to which word might be *le mot juste* in that particular context. In many instances the related words are synonymous, but don't count on it.

The most famous of thesaurus-makers, the English physician Peter Mark Roget (1779–1869), was the fortunate author of the *Thesaurus of English Words and Phrases*, which was printed in 28 editions in his lifetime alone. Roget, a scholar who helped to found the University of London, would no doubt have been enormously pleased to know that his name has been perpetuated in any number of works (some worthy and some not).

Anyone who so desires may use the name Roget to publish a thesaurus, now that the right to use it has passed into the public domain. The same is true of the name Webster, as in "dictionary."

Therefore, readers of these kinds of works should use caution in purchasing them. Don't buy them on the strength of the honored name in the title. Look at them carefully for quality and accuracy, and for the uses *you* would put them to. Ask a respected librarian, editor, or writer for the names of the best books of those kinds.

DESCRIPTIVE AND "PRESCRIPTIVE" DICTIONARIES

Many innocents believe that if a word appears in a dictionary it is prima facie correct. People who wouldn't dream of using "ain't" may draw the wrong conclusion from its mere appearance in good dictionaries unless they read the entire entry carefully.

Dictionaries of the English language are descriptive—that is, they describe usage as it *is*, not necessarily as it should be. The best ones have usage notes that are invaluable to the serious writer: When questionable words are entered, they are described as colloquial, nonstandard, dialectical, regional, or jocular. Non-American speakers as well are thus enabled to draw the proper conclusions.

There are no prescriptive dictionaries of the English language. If they are "prescriptive," they are by definition books on usage. Of course, the usage books may be arranged in dictionary style, that is, alphabetically.

In the editorial offices of dictionaries sit dozens of editors, scanning newspapers, magazines, journals, and books for suitable entries in the next editions of their monumental and endlessly fascinating books. They listen to speakers in person and by means of radio and television, wherever English is spoken. Each entry and its etymology are painstakingly documented; dinosaur tracks are not more carefully examined. Words and phrases qualify for entrance into the dictionary when a sufficient number of sightings are recorded.

You and I are contributing in our small way to this noble endeavor.

BOOKS ON USAGE

When questions of usage arise, consult the books on usage. Dictionaries are not made for that purpose.

Words are abstractions, symbols. They are not palpable or tangible except as they appear on paper. They are flighty creatures. They break upon the consciousness like waves, billions of them flashing like St. Elmo's fire across the brain in a second. Some remain on the strand like beached whales, impossible to dispose of.

Being insubstantial, words are helpless to defend themselves. They must rely on the judgment of users. Customs change, the culture changes, the character of a nation changes, and usage changes with them. There is no "right" or "wrong" in usage. There is only consensus—the consensus of the good writers and speakers of English.

Writers, editors, and speakers are continuously engaged in setting usage, whether they know it or not. But they're not the only ones. Yogi Berra and Dizzy Dean are as likely to be quoted as are Bertrand Russell, Morris R. Cohen, and Joseph Conrad.

Books on usage serve many purposes. Above all, they save time and obviate the acrimony of disputes.

CHAPTER 20

Word Origins, Oddities, and Stories

Technical, scientific, medical, and other lexicons contain words that are exactly the same in English as in the original Latin or Greek. Some terms are either Latin or Greek, but others are hybrids—practical mixtures of those languages.

Cardiopulmonary is such a word. The *cardio* part comes from the Greek *kardia*, heart; the *pulmonary* part comes from the Latin *pulmo*, lung.

Perinatal, referring to the period just before, during, and after birth, is another such word. *Peri-* is from the Greek, around; *natal* is from the Latin *natus*, born. This *natal* should not be confused with the other *natal*, from the Latin *natis*, meaning the rump or buttock (usually used in the plural—*nates*, the buttocks). Neither should it be confused with *natatory*, which has to do with swimming rather than birth or the buttocks.

A-, AN-

A- or *an-* is a privative or antonymous prefix (a prefix that changes the sense of a word from positive to negative). The antonymous *a-* is used in such words as *atheist* (Greek *theos*, "god") and *asexual*. In elements beginning with h (usually of Greek or Latin origin), *an-* is used instead of *a-*: *anhydrous*. The antonymous prefix *an-* is also seen in such words as *anodyne* (Greek odyne, "pain").

The spatial preposition *ana* (Greek for "up") becomes a prefix and a combining form, as in *anabolism* (from Greek *anabole*, a rising up); *an-* (from *ana*) is also an assimilated or elided combining form: *anode* (Greek *anodos*, a way up, from *ana*, up, and *hodos*, way).

The antonymous prefix *an-* is analogous to the antonymous prefixes *in-* and *un-*.

ADVANTAGE OF PUBLISHING IN ENGLISH

If Nicolas C. Paulesco, a researcher in Romania, had published the results of his work in English instead of Romanian, he probably would have received a Nobel prize. Instead, Banting and Macleod received the 1923 Nobel Prize in Physiology or Medicine for their isolation in 1921, together with Best and Collip, of a hormone (later called insulin) from the pancreas.

Paulesco's articles on the subject, published in 1921 in *Comptes Rendus des Séances de la Société de Biologie et de ses Filiales* (Paris) (Vol. 85, part 2) and other French journals, dealt with his isolation of pancreatic extracts and the physiologic effects of insulin.

The term insulin (Latin *insula*, island) was taken by the Canadian group from the islets of Langerhans, whose beta cells secrete insulin in the pancreas.

BEDLAM

Bedlam is from the popular name for the Hospital of St. Mary of Bethlehem in London, a hospital for the mentally ill. It stems from Middle English *Bedlem* or *Bethlem*, an alternative spelling of Bethlehem.

CABAL

The following *acrostic* comes from the initials of the last names of advisers to Charles II of England:

Clifford
Ashley
Buckingham
Arlington
Lauderdale

However, this acrostic is not the origin of the word *cabal*.

Cabal is not an acronym. It is a clandestine group or organization; the word comes from ancient Hebrew, so that it considerably antedates Charles II and his kitchen cabinet.

CACOGRAPHY

Orthography, in its specific meaning of correct spelling, has an antonym: *cacography*.

SUB ROSA

This Latin phrase, meaning literally "under the rose," has an obscure origin. Mythology tells us that Cupid gave a rose to Harpocrates, the god of silence, as a bribe to keep secret the amorous adventures of Venus. The rose became the symbol of discretion and silence; it was carved on the walls or ceilings of banqueting halls as a reminder to the guests that "what was spoken *sub vino* [under the influence of wine] was not to be repeated *sub divo* [in the open air]. In the 16th century it was placed over confessionals" (*Brewer's Dictionary of Phrase and Fable*).

CAESAREA LEX

Lex is Latin for law; *caesarea* is its modifying adjective meaning caesarean. Since this law undoubtedly predates the birth of Gaius Julius Caesar by centuries, the adjective is written with a lowercase *c*.

This Roman law stated that if a woman who was about to give birth died in the process, the child would nonetheless be delivered alive—if possible—by caesarean section.

(See the entry "Cesarean, Caesarean, cesarean, or caesarean?" in Chapter 4, "Medical and Pharmaceutical Pointers," which explains more fully why the term for this surgical procedure is written with an initial lowercase *c*.)

A CHANGE IN DIAGNOSIS

One can sympathize (or empathize) with the diagnostician, who has the task of correlating the patient's subjective complaints with objective observations.

Consider the situation faced by this physician. A booklet published by the British Medical Association, "You and Your Guts," describes the case of a middle-aged woman who complained that she could not swallow properly. After examining her throat and related regions, he told her, "Madam, it is the change"—meaning menopause. He was wrong, though correct. She had swallowed some coins, change given to her when shopping.

That's the end of the story as I received it. I don't know how the medical (or surgical) problem was resolved.

CIRCADIAN

This term was coined in 1959 by Franz Halberg, of the University of Minnesota, from Latin *circa*, "about," and *dies*, "day." It means "about a day," and is used to refer to the internal "daily" rhythm of animals and plants.

Thus was born a good neologism.

"DESIGNER DRUG"

A Nebraska man was found not guilty of a charge of making and distributing a "designer drug" known as "ecstasy" because the chemical name of the drug, methylenedioxymethamphetamine, was misspelled in a state law.

> Designer drugs are synthetic substances that closely resemble, in structure and effects produced, the particular drugs that are strictly controlled in the United States. These drugs are "designed" to take advantage of American drug laws that have not specifically prohibited their manufacture and use.

The definition is from *Drugs and Drug Abuse: A Reference Text*.

The defense attorney contended that factors other than the misspelling had contributed to the "not guilty" finding and that the state had not proved that the drug was illegal.

The judge's verdict was based on the finding that the Nebraskan had not violated the law—he did not possess the drug named in the law.

I foresee a new profession—editors for legislators.

ENGLISH VS. GREEK AND LATIN

One can understand why, in some instances, a single word is used, although it may seem pretentious:

Dyslogia. This is a fancy word meaning impairment of the power of reasoning, leading to difficulty in expressing ideas through speech.

Hellenomania. The American Psychiatric Association's *Psychiatric Glossary* defined *hellenomania* as the tendency to use unwieldy Latin or Greek expressions instead of immediately understandable English terms. The definition goes on to say that this term "characterizes the pseudoerudite jargon of many fields." So true.

Lethologica. If you forget your best friend's name when introducing her or him, you are suffering from lethologica, the inability (usually transient) to remember a name, term, or proper noun.

Don't bother looking up these last two words in *Webster III*; they're not entered.

Some sufferers are frustrated not only by lethologica but also by "staircase wisdom," the wonderfully descriptive term (*esprit de l'escalier* in French) for the stinging retort you think of *after* a confrontation with a snob at the cocktail party.

Examples of repartee you think of *during* these episodes:

Oh yeah?
So's your old man!

Examples of repartee you think of afterward:

And you, madam, are ugly. But I shall be sober in the morning.
Oh yeah? Well, we also serve who only punctuate.
I never forget a face, but in your case I'll make an exception.
That's not writing, that's typing.
(To a thin man) Sir, you are like a pin, but without either its head or its point.
If you had it all over again, would you fall in love with yourself?
Play us a medley of your hit.
You have van Gogh's ear for music.

FISTMELE

Fistmele, from *fist* plus *mele*, an obsolete variant of *meal* (measure), is defined in *Webster III* as the breadth of a fist with thumb stuck out, used especially in archery to give the height of a string from a braced bow: about 7 inches.

Painters (artists) and film directors use this movement.

SYCOSIS

Despite the similarity in pronunciation, this word has absolutely nothing in common with a psychiatric and psychologic term—psychosis.

Sycosis is—plain and simple—barber's itch. The full term is *sycosis barbae* (vulgaris).

FOIBLE

This word comes from the French *faible*, weak (you can see where our *feeble* comes from). It means a shortcoming or small flaw. Aside from that, it means the part of a sword blade or foil blade between the middle and the point, as opposed to *forte*, the strong part of the sword, between the middle and the hilt.

That *forte* is French, so it's pronounced as if it were spelled fort (in English), and is not to be confused with the Italian *forte*, a two-syllable musical term that means loud.

HIBERNATION AND ESTIVATION

Everyone knows what *hibernation* means—bears, for instance, hibernate all winter and emerge in the spring from their caves.

Zoologists know that *estivation* is the state of dormancy or torpor during the summer—a state shared by snails, crabs, and seashore visitors.

IN-, IN-

One kind of *in-* is a spatial prefix, meaning in, on, or into, as in such Latin-derived words as *insurrection* (from *surrectus*, the past participle of *surgere*, to rise), *inflammable* (from *flamma*, flame), *induration* (*durare*, to harden), *improvise* (*provisus*, the past participle of *providere*, to foresee or anticipate), *information* (*formare*, to form or shape), *innovation* (*novare*, to alter or make new), and *injection* (*jacere*, to throw).

Another kind of *in-* is an antonymous or privative prefix, as in *insensitive* (from *sensus, senso*, perception), *immature* (from *maturus*, ripe), *illegible* (from *legibilis*, capable of being read), *impossible* (from *possibilis*, from *posse*, to be able), *injury* (from *jus, juris*, right, justice), or *irreverent* (from *revereri*, to stand in awe of).

The suffix *-less* is a privative suffix.

In consonance with the perpetual move in language toward ease of pronunciation and euphony, the prefix *in-* changes (is assimilated or elided) to *il-, im-,* or *ir-* to match the first letter of the next syllable: *illegal, immoral, irreducible.*

JANUS WORDS

These are double-faced or double-headed words—words that have opposite meanings. The term "Janus" comes from the Roman god who was the keeper of portals and the patron of beginnings and endings. His statues show him as having two faces, one in the front of his head and the other at the back, symbolizing his power to see both the beginning and the end of everything.

The first month in our calendar, January, is named after him, since it represents the beginning of the new year.

My short list of Janus words follows. Let me know if you have others.

bone	priceless
cleave	ravel
invaluable	sanction
let	seed
oversight	

To bone is to build or provide bone and also to remove bone.

To cleave is to cut asunder and also to cling to.

Invaluable means precious, as in gems, and also means without value.

Let implies permission. In another context, it means an obstacle, impediment. Tennis players know that *let* means a stroke or point that has to be replayed. The phrase "without let or hindrance" is seldom used outside a legal context.

Let is actually two different words, from different roots. It has both a "permission" sense (the transitive verb) and a "hindrance" sense (the noun). In the duel scene in the Shakespeare play *Hamlet*, the prince exclaims, "By Heaven! I'll make a ghost of him that lets me." That's the original wording. However, in Sir Laurence Olivier's film production, the prince exclaims, "By Heaven! I'll make a ghost of him that hinders me." Olivier wanted everyone to understand and enjoy Shakespeare. Undoubtedly he figured that few modern viewers would know the meaning of "let" as Shakespeare used it, so he took the liberty of changing one word. He could do that because he produced the film and starred in it. A talented man indeed.

An *oversight* is something that is overlooked. *Oversight* is the noun one thinks of in connection with "overseeing."

Priceless means valuable and also means without price.

To ravel means the same as to unravel: to loosen threads.

To sanction a process means to approve it. However, *sanctions*, usually business, financial or industrial, against a nation are intended to have unfavorable consequences.

One plants a garden by *seeding* it. One *seeds* an apple by removing the seeds.

LINGUA FRANCA

English is spoken as a national language in more countries and over a larger area than any other language. It is the leading candidate for world language, and is in fact the *lingua franca*, the language of commerce and trade throughout the world.

A *lingua franca* (plural, *lingua francas* or *linguae francae*) is a common—hybrid or pidgin—language (originally Italian intermixed with Arabic, Greek, French, and Spanish) that is used for ease of communication among peoples who speak different languages. *Lingua franca* in Italian means literally "Frankish language."

Frankish is an early Germanic language that was spoken in an area that is now France, where some language vestiges of the Franks' occupation of Gaul in the third century can still be seen.

NOR-

At one time the prefix *nor-*, as in norepinephrine (noradrenalin), was a partial acronym meaning "nitrogen without radical," from the German *Nitrogen ohne Radikal*.

Nor- is now used more broadly as a chemical prefix in a number of chemical compounds. Consult your medical dictionary or pharmacology text for specific information.

AND THE REST IS HISTORY

Words are the most powerful things on earth. They can hurt—they can heal—and they can cause wars.

A battle of the Crimean War (1853–1856) on October 25, 1854, might have turned out differently if an order of the British general had not been misinterpreted.

Earlier in the day, the British troops had repulsed the Russian forces at Balaklava in the Crimea, a peninsula in southern Russia. Pressing the advantage, Lord Cardigan gave the command to "charge the guns." His shouted order—probably intended to mean to load the guns with powder—was misunderstood in the general confusion.

In the battle that followed, the cavalry brigade of some 670 Englishmen attacked a virtually impregnable Russian position. More than two thirds of Cardigan's men were killed or wounded.

Alfred Lord Tennyson immortalized this tragedy of war and words in *The Charge of the Light Brigade*:

> Someone had blundered ✻ ✻ ✻
> Into the jaws of death,
> Into the mouth of hell
> Rode the six hundred.

Three eponymous terms for garments came out of this battle for Sevastopol.

Lord (Baron) Raglan, the commanding officer of the British troops, gave his name to an overcoat with sleeves that go to the shoulders without shoulder seams. I conjecture that the coat was custom-made for him—he had lost his sword arm at Waterloo.

Lord (Earl) Cardigan led the cavalry charge on the fateful day and was the first man to reach the Russian lines. The cardigan, a sweater that buttons down the front instead of being pulled over the head, is named for him.

The Balaklava helmet is a close-fitting wool hood.

NUDE MICE

That's not a joke or a typo. They exist.

Not only is hair, or fur, missing—the thymus gland is missing as well, so that certain lymphocytes have no chance to develop. Nude mice are used in cancer research because cancer cells of humans proliferate experimentally in the mutants under conditions closely resembling those in humans.

The athymic mouse mutant was first noticed by J. H. Isaacson and B. M. Cattanach (reported in 1962) because of the absence of fur.

The thymusless mouse is the first discrete animal model of a severe immunodeficiency resulting from the lack of a thymus and the ensuing T lymphocyte defect.

These mice do not ordinarily reject transplanted organs or skin grafts. Researchers treat them with experimental antineoplastic drugs or agents to see whether these substances might be effective in humans as well.

Athymic mouse mutants are inordinately vulnerable to disease; their environment must therefore be kept absolutely sterile and free of pollutants and contaminants, particularly the organism that causes murine hepatitis.

The mutation, which was detected by N. A. Grist, occurred at the Virus Laboratories, Ruchill Hospital, Glasgow, Scotland, in a closed but not inbred stock of albino mice. He sent nude and phenotypically normal mice from the same litter to the Institute of Animal Genetics in Edinburgh.

The genetics were first described in detail in 1966 by S. P. Flanagan, who gave the name "nude, genetic symbol *nu*" to the athymic mouse mutants. His most notable findings about these mice were the reduction in body growth and an extreme reduction in life span: 45 percent of them died within 2 weeks of birth, and all of them died within 25 weeks. There was a high incidence of massive parenchymal necrosis of the liver in the dead mice.

Researchers hope that the early studies can be used as a model for the study of other mutants. The *nu* gene has been transferred to strains of inbred mice.

The Nude Mouse Secretariat in Copenhagen maintains a registry of human malignant tumors that have been transplanted into the athymic mouse mutants.

OCTOTHORP

Octothorp is the name for the "number" symbol, the "pound" symbol on your pushbutton telephone, or the tic-tac-toe symbol (the game is also known as "noughts and crosses"). Musicians know a variant as the "sharp" symbol, as in C# minor; editors and proofreaders use it to mark a (hairline) space; and computer users call it a crunch. In still other fields it is known as a crosshatch or hatchmark.

Here's an irresistible story, as you will see from the following extracts of a letter that Frederick C. Mish, Ph.D., Editorial Director at Merriam-Webster Inc., Springfield, Mass., wrote to me in 1986. It is here published with his gracious permission:

> This is the substance of a letter on the supposed origin of *octothorp* . . . The letter is from an employee of Bell Canada, who had it from another employee of Bell Canada, who was on loan to AT&T in New York at the time. The latter did not coin the word himself but knew the people who did. So this story is third- or fourth-hand to you, fourth- or fifth- to your readers. You see why we lexicographers tend to be skeptical of these reports. Nonetheless, it is a good story, and here it is:
>
> The term "octotherp" was invented by three people . . . who, about 1965, were in the marketing section of AT&T in New York City. One afternoon during a discussion over coffee, these gentlemen noted that the # *symbol* had no name, not even in the printing trade, and felt that it should be given a name. But what kind of name would be suitable?
>
> These gentlemen looked at the # symbol and noted that there are 8 points and 8 spaces around the symbol—hence the term "octo" for 8. Then came the task of finding something to go behind the "octo." They were looking for something that had a good solid end; this would be the letter "p," which in the English language is a very strong ending for any word. The "th" came about by the desire for [a sound that may be unique to the English language]. Our heroes were trying to figure out how to connect the "th" with the "p" when apparently someone belched. This gave them the idea of "erp," then "therp," and so the word "octotherp." Because it was a name that was new, it caught on.
>
> Some people began calling the word "octothorp" instead of "octotherp" because they could not imagine what "therp" is. . . . In . . . England there are a number of villages, etc., whose name ends in "thorpe," such as Scunthorpe. (A linguist at McGill University in Montreal once suggested that "octothorp" meant 8 villages.) The name gradually came into wider use within AT&T and elsewhere, but as "octothorp," not "octotherp."
>
> The etymology given in the 1986 Addenda Section of *Webster's Third New International Dictionary* is [*octo* + *thorp*, of unknown origin; fr. the eight points on its circumference]. That is as far as we would care to go in the present state of our knowledge.

ORCHIDECTOMY

For readers who are not conversant with medical terminology, *orchidectomy* is not a cutting or grafting of orchids but removal of the testes or a testis.

The alternative term is *orchiectomy*.

This example illustrates the hazards of folk (fake) etymology.

TETRALOGY

While a novel of Isaac Asimov's was in press, he and the publisher contemplated using a slogan on the dust jacket, "The fourth book in The Foundation trilogy." Hugh O'Neill, the editor of the book, said, "Only in the world of sci-fi could you have four in a trilogy. But then we were afraid people wouldn't get the joke."

So, although the publisher's catalogue included the original slogan, the new baby (*Foundation's Edge*) became on the dust jacket the fourth book in the "series."

OXYMORONS

The word *oxymoron* is itself an oxymoron. It comes from the Greek *oxys*, sharp, plus *moron*, dull.

Here are a few oxymorons, some home-made and the others cribbed:

bad grammar	deafening silence
child psychiatrist	disorganized system
conspicuous absence	favorite disease
criminal lawyer	giant minimarket
critical acclaim (a pun as well)	guest host
	jumbo shrimp
cruel kindness	killing kindness

There are cynics who offend a goodly portion of the population by maintaining that these are oxymorons also:

business ethics
military intelligence

PANDEMONIUM

This utilitarian lowercase word is from Pandaemonium, the capital of Hell in John Milton's *Paradise Lost*. It comes from the Greek *pan* (meaning "all") and *daemonium* ("evil spirit").

POUND

Why is *pound* abbreviated *lb.* or *lb*? The English word *pound* comes from the Latin *pondo*, weight. Originally the Latin phrase was *libra pondo*, pound in weight.

Since *lb.* is itself an abbreviation, no terminal *s* is necessary:

The device weighed 12 lb.

The British pound sterling was originally silver weighing one pound. Its symbol, £, reflects the *l* in *libra*.

RICHTER SCALE

Although these facts are hardly world-shaking, I find them interesting enough to recount.

In 1935 the seismologist Charles F. Richter, of the California Institute of Technology, devised a logarithmic (and therefore theoretically open-ended or infinite) scale ranging from 0 to 9 to measure the amount of energy released by earthquakes. Each point in the scale represents a magnitude ten times as great as the preceding number. A number 7 earthquake, therefore, would be 10 times as strong as a quake of the magnitude of 6.

So far no earthquake has been recorded with a Richter number of 9. Seismologists have calculated that the disastrous San Francisco earthquake in 1906 would have registered 8.3 on the Richter scale, had the scale existed at that time. The 1964 earthquake in Anchorage, Alaska, measured 8.4 on the Richter scale.

The October 17, 1989, earthquake in the San Francisco Bay area registered 7.1 on the Richter scale and probably at least 7.0 on the Mercalli scale. For seismophiles and numerophiles, the epicenter of what is officially named (by the U.S. Geological Survey) the Loma Prieta earthquake was latitude 37.036°N and longitude 121.883°W; the depth was 19 kilometers.

The Italian seismologist Giuseppe Mercalli (1850–1914) devised a scale that measures the damage caused by the energy earthquakes release. Damage is still the main criterion in assessing the effects of an earthquake on the region and the population.

HIROSHIMA AND NAGASAKI

In *Native Tongues,* Charles Berlitz (yes, of that extraordinary family) describes several fascinating "Language Incidents That Changed History," including the story about a mistranslation of *mokusatsu*, a Japanese word that can mean "ignore," "have no comment," or "withhold comment."

Hiroshima and Nagasaki might still be standing in their original forms if *mokusatsu* had been translated differently. Before the United States Air Force dropped the first atom bomb, the government warned Japan of a terrible new weapon and offered that government the opportunity of surrendering to avoid destruction of its cities. The Imperial Government announced that it was following a policy of *mokusatsu* until the cabinet could consider and act on the offer. "This verb was translated as 'ignore'—and the Bomb was dropped."

When Berlitz first started to speak as a child, he learned four languages at the same time. In his preface to the 1982 edition, this prodigious man, who up to that time had acquired about 28 languages, wrote:

> For language, reinforced and immortalized through writing, has been the most important development in the progress of the human species, leading it from family group barbarism, not unlike animal packs, to its present dominion of the earth and a force toward the exploration of the cosmos.

SOLECISM

This word, meaning a syntactical or grammatical error, is from the Greek *soloikismos*. *Soloikos*, its root, means speaking incorrectly. A corrupt form of Attic was spoken by colonists in Soloi, a city in ancient Cilicia.

Solecism also means an absurdity; it can even mean a breach of propriety in decorum or etiquette or an incongruity in logic or facts.

STRANGE DISORDERS

Many strange disorders, thitherto unreported in the literature, have been described, most prominently in the *New England Journal of Medicine*.

Since these conditions are anomalous, some may be of the tongue-in-cheek variety.

> *Back-pocket sciatica*: a disorder caused by pressure on the sciatic nerve in the gluteus maximus, brought about by a bulging wallet in the back pocket.
>
> *Congestive fart failure*: gastrointestinal unease, caused by bloating and gas pains, characterized by difficulty in expelling the cause of the malaise.
>
> *Disco felon*: fulminating infection of a finger, caused by excessive snapping of the fingers while disco dancing.
>
> *Jeans folliculitis*: irritation or inflammation of the hair follicles around the upper thighs, caused by wearing excessively tight jeans or dungarees.

Ponderous-purse disease: pain in the neck, shoulder, and upper torso, caused by inappropriately heavy shoulder purses.

Proofreader's prostatitis: an occupational disorder suffered by the proofreader at a pornographic publishing house.

Slot-machine tendinitis: pain in the shoulder, frequently seen in visitors to Las Vegas or Atlantic City.

Space-Invaders' wrist: pain in the wrist brought on by excessive playing of a popular video game.

UNITED NATIONS CONTRETEMPS

During the Cold War, in 1976 to be exact, a particularly nasty incident occurred in the United Nations Security Council, when the Soviet representative, Yakov Malik, charged that Americans were trying to twist the Soviet position on colonial issues. He admonished Americans to "take care" (as the interpreter translated it) in describing Soviet policies.

The United States representative, Daniel Patrick Moynihan, snapped that Americans didn't "give a damn" about Soviet threats. Later, Malik complained that his words had been mistranslated and misinterpreted. He had said "take heed," not "take care."

Although these two phrases seem almost interchangeable, in this rancorous political context "take heed" has a more moderate connotation than "take care," which seems to carry a threat or warning.

STUDENT t-TEST

Some house styles prescribe italicization of *t* in this context, and some don't use the hyphen.

William S. Gossett (1876–1937), a statistician with the Guinness brewery in Dublin, Ireland, empirically derived a statistical quantity having to do with large-sample experiments. Because Guinness forbade the publication of research findings by its employees, Gossett sent the report of his findings to Karl Pearson, who had been his teacher.

Beginning in 1908, Gossett's research results were published under the pseudonym "Student" (not, as some think, "A. Student") in the journal *Biometrika*, of which Pearson, happily for the coming generations of statisticians (and Gossett), was the Editor.

The article, titled "The Probable Error of a Mean," was published by "Student" in Volume 6, No. 1 (March 1908) of *Biometrika*.

Karl Pearson is generally considered the father of the modern science of statistics. Professor E. S. Pearson, also a world-famous statistician, is his son.

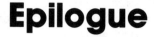

Epilogue

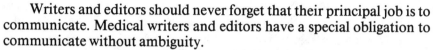

Writers and editors should never forget that their principal job is to communicate. Medical writers and editors have a special obligation to communicate without ambiguity.

There are few Lewis Thomases and Sir William Oslers among us. Nonetheless, we write because we must: some because of an inner urge—fire in the belly; some because of the urge to share medical knowledge and experiences; some because of the "publish or perish" requirement of academia; some because they want to make a living at it.

If you have something to say, write it. Share it with the world. Don't use the excuse that "everything has already been said—and well." No one else can say it quite the way you would.

If you are an editor, resist the temptation to paraphrase an already perfect sentence, simply because you think your version would sound more learned. Don't say "The Divine Being donateth and the Divine Being deleteth" when you mean "the Lord giveth and the Lord taketh away."

The written word is a communication forever. It enables those who come after us to utilize the wisdom we have so painfully—and gainfully—acquired. The written word is our connection with the past and our bridge to the future.

Henry van Dyke (1852–1933) was an American minister, poet, and essayist. In an extraordinarily inspirational message, he wrote:

> Use what talents you possess. The woods would be very silent if no birds sang there except those that sang best.

The writing of this book has been one of the great ventures of my life. I love the language, and its proper use has become one of my passions. My ruling passion is the pursuit of excellence.

One reason I undertook this arduous task was to put into book form my opinions and preferences about usage—some of the things I've learned in a long editing and writing career.

Another reason was my desire to carry further a splendid endeavor: preserving the beauty and utility of the English language.

In his inimitably witty, succinct manner, Theodore M. Bernstein wrote what has become my favorite quotation and the motto on my shield; I have rendered the second part of it into Latin as *Acumina sanguinem mittere possunt*:

> This may seem like a fine point,
> but fine points can draw blood.

Never stop learning.

Bibliography

The following is a representative list of books consulted in the preparation of this book. There may be later editions of some.

Asimov, I.: *Biographical Encyclopedia of Science and Technology*, rev. ed. New York, Avon, 1976.

Barzun, J.: *On Writing, Editing, and Publishing*. Chicago, University of Chicago Press, 1971.

———: *A Word or Two Before You Go . . .: Brief Essays on Language.* Middletown, Conn.: Wesleyan University Press, 1986.

Beck, E.M. (ed.): *Familiar Quotations by John Bartlett*, 14th ed. rev. and enlarged. Boston, Little, Brown, 1968.

Berkow, R., et al. (eds.): *The Merck Manual*, 15th ed. Rahway, N.J., Merck & Co., 1987.

Berlitz, C.: *Native Tongues.* New York, Putnam, 1982.

Bernstein, T.M.: *The Careful Writer: A Modern Guide to English Usage.* New York, Atheneum, 1965.

———: *Dos, Don'ts & Maybes of English Usage.* New York, Times Books, 1977.

———: *Miss Thistlebottom's Hobgoblins: The Careful Writer's Guide to the Taboos, Bugbears and Outmoded Rules of English Usage.* New York, Farrar, Straus and Giroux, 1971.

———: *Watch Your Language.* Great Neck, N.Y., Channel, 1958.

Billups, N.; Billups, S.: *American Drug Index.* Philadelphia, J.B. Lippincott, 1990.

Braunwald, E. (ed.): *Harrison's Principles of Internal Medicine*, 11th ed. New York, McGraw-Hill, 1987.

Buchanan, R.E.; Gibbons, N.E. (eds.): *Bergey's Manual of Determinative Bacteriology*, 8th ed. Baltimore, Williams & Wilkins, 1974.

Buchanan-Brown, J., et al. (eds.): *Le Mot Juste.* New York, Random House, 1981.

Budavari, S., et al. (eds.): *The Merck Index*, 11th ed. Rahway, N.J., Merck & Co., 1989.

Bulfinch, T.: *The Age of Fable, or Beauties of Mythology.* New York, New American Library, 1962.

Burchfield, R.: *The English Language*. New York, Oxford University Press, 1986.

CBE Style Manual Committee: *CBE Style Manual*, 5th ed. rev. and expanded. Bethesda, Md., Council of Biology Editors, 1983.

Charlton, J.: *The Writer's Quotation Book*. New York, Penguin, 1985.

The Chicago Manual of Style, 13th ed. rev. and expanded. Chicago, University of Chicago Press, 1982.

Clemente, C.D.: *Anatomy: A Regional Atlas of the Human Body*, 3rd ed. Baltimore, Urban & Schwarzenberg, 1987.

Curme, G.O.: *English Grammar*. New York, Barnes & Noble, 1947.

Davis, N.K.; Cohen, M.R.: *Medication Errors: Causes and Prevention*. Philadelphia, George F. Stickley, 1981.

Day, R.A.: *How to Write and Publish a Scientific Paper*, 3rd ed. Phoenix Ariz., Oryx Press, 1988.

DeBakey, L.: *The Scientific Journal: Editorial Policies and Practices: Guidelines for Editors, Reviewers, and Authors*. St. Louis, C.V. Mosby, 1976.

Dutch R.A. (ed.): *The St. Martin's Roget's Thesaurus of English Words and Phrases*. New York, St. Martin's Press, 1965.

Ebbitt, W.R.; Ebbitt, D.R.: *Writer's Guide and Index to English*, 7th ed. Glenview, Ill., Scott, Foresman, 1982.

Evans, B.: *Dictionary of Mythology, Mainly Classical*. New York, Dell, 1970.

Evans, B.; Evans, C.: *A Dictionary of Contemporary American Usage*. New York, Random House, 1957.

Evans, I.H.: *Brewer's Dictionary of Phrase and Fable*, 14th ed. New York, Harper & Row, 1989.

Fitzhenry, R.I. (ed.): *Barnes & Noble Book of Quotations*, rev. and enlarged. New York, Barnes & Noble, 1987.

Follett, W.: *Modern American Usage*. New York, Hill & Wang, 1966.

Garb, S.; Krakauer, E.; Justice, C.: *Abbreviations and Acronyms in Medicine and Nursing*. New York, Springer, 1976.

Goodman, L.S.; Gilman, A. (eds.): *The Pharmacological Basis of Therapeutics*, 8th ed. New York, Pergamon, 1990.

Goodwin, R.A.; Flexner, S. (eds.): *March's Thesaurus and Dictionary of the English Language*. New York, Abbeville, 1980.

Gove, P.B. (ed.): *Webster's Third New International Dictionary of the English Language, Unabridged*. Springfield, Mass., G. & C. Merriam, 1981.

Gowers, E.: *The Complete Plain Words*. Baltimore, Penguin, 1962.

Graves, R.; Hodge, A.: *The Reader over Your Shoulder*. New York, Collier, 1966.

Griffiths, M.C. (ed.): *USAN and the USP Dictionary of Drug Names*. Rockville, Md., United States Pharmacopeial Convention, 1989.

Hamilton, B.; Guidos, B. (eds.): *MASA: Medical Acronyms, Symbols & Abbreviations*. New York, Neal-Schuman, 1984.

Hamilton, E.: *Mythology*. New York, New American Library, 1969.

Harris, W.H.; Levey, J.S. (eds.): *The New Columbia Encyclopedia*. New York, Columbia University Press, 1975 (distributed by J.B. Lippincott).

Haubrich, W.S.: *Medical Meanings: A Glossary of Word Origins*. New York, Harcourt Brace Jovanovich, 1984.

Hollinshead, H.: *Textbook of Anatomy*, 4th ed. Philadelphia, Harper & Row, 1985.

Hopper, V.F., et al. (eds.): *Barron's Essentials of English*, 3rd ed. New York, Barron's Educational Series, 1982.

Horowitz, L.: *Knowing Where to Look: The Ultimate Guide to Research*. Cincinnati, Writer's Digest Books, 1984.

Huth, E.J.: *How to Write and Publish Papers in the Medical Sciences*. Philadelphia, ISI Press, 1982.

———: *Medical Style & Format: An International Manual for Authors, Editors, and Publishers*. Philadelphia, ISI Press, 1987.

Iverson, C., et al. (eds.): *American Medical Association Manual of Style*, 8th ed. Baltimore, Williams & Wilkins, 1989.

Jablonski, S.: *Illustrated Dictionary of Eponymic Syndromes and Diseases and Their Synonyms*. Philadelphia, W.B. Saunders, 1969.

Jacobs, M.R.; Fehr, K.O'B. (revisers): *Drugs and Drug Abuse*. Toronto, Addiction Research Foundation, 1987.

Jordan, L. (ed.): *The New York Times Manual of Style and Usage*. New York, Times Books, 1976.

King, L.: *Why Not Say It Clearly*. Boston, Little, Brown, 1978.

Lentner, M.: *Elementary Applied Statistics*. Tarrytown-on-Hudson, N.Y., Bogden & Quigley, 1972.

Lloyd, S.M. (ed.): *The Penguin Roget's Thesaurus of English Words and Phrases*. New York, Penguin, 1985.

Logan, C.M.; Rice, M.K. (eds.): *Logan's Medical and Scientific Abbreviations*. Philadelphia, J.B. Lippincott, 1987.

Macmillan Dictionary of Quotations. New York, Macmillan, 1989.

Magalini S.I.; Scrascia, E.: *Dictionary of Medical Syndromes*, 2nd ed. Philadelphia, J.B. Lippincott, 1981.

Maggio, R.: *The Nonsexist Word Finder: A Dictionary of Gender-Free Usage*. Phoenix, Ariz., Oryx Press, 1987.

Mallery, R.D.: *Grammar, Rhetoric and Composition for Home Study*. New York, Barnes & Noble, 1970.

Mawson C.O.S.: *Dictionary of Foreign Terms*, 2nd ed. New York, Crowell, 1974.

Miller, M.; Swift, K: *The Handbook of Nonsexist Writing*. New York, Harper & Row (Barnes & Noble Books), 1980.

Mish, F.C. (ed.): *Webster's Ninth New Collegiate Dictionary*. Springfield, Mass., Merriam-Webster, 1983.

——— (ed.): *Webster's Word Histories*. Springfield, Mass., Merriam-Webster, 1989.

Mitchell, R.: *Less than Words Can Say*. Boston, Little, Brown, 1979.

Morris, W. (ed.): *The American Heritage Dictionary of the English Language.* New York, American Heritage Publishing Co., 1969.

Neilson, W.A. (ed.): *Webster's Biographical Dictionary.* Springfield, Mass., G. & C. Merriam, 1976.

Newman, E.: *Strictly Speaking.* Indianapolis, Bobbs-Merrill, 1974.

Nicholson, M.: *A Dictionary of American-English Usage* (based on Fowler's *Modern English Usage*). New York, Oxford University Press, 1957.

Nurnberg, M: *I Always Look Up the Word "E•gre•gious."* Englewood Cliffs, N.J., Prentice-Hall, 1981.

Opdycke, J.B.: *Harper's English Grammar.* New York, Harper & Row (Warner Books ed.), 1965.

Partridge, E.: *The Concise Usage and Abusage.* New York, Philosophical Library, 1955.

Physicians' Desk Reference, 44th ed. Oradell, N.J., Medical Economics Company, 1990.

Room, A.: *The Penguin Dictionary of Confusibles.* New York, Penguin, 1979.

Silver, D.J.: *A History of Judaism.* Vol. 1, *From Abraham to Maimonides.* New York, Basic Books, 1974.

Simpson, D.P.: *Cassell's New Latin Dictionary.* New York, Funk & Wagnalls, 1968.

Simpson, J.D.: *Simpson's Contemporary Quotations.* Boston, Houghton Mifflin, 1988.

Skillin, M.E.; Gay, R.M.: *Words into Type,* 3rd ed. rev. Englewood Cliffs, N.J., Prentice-Hall, 1974.

Sledd, J.; Ebbitt, W.R. (eds.): *Dictionaries and* That *Dictionary.* Chicago, Scott, Foresman, 1962.

Stedman's Medical Dictionary, 24th ed. Baltimore, Williams & Wilkins, 1982.

Strunk, W., Jr.; White, E.B.: *The Elements of Style.* New York, Macmillan, 1959.

Taylor E.J.; Anderson D.M.; Patwell J.M., et al.: *Dorland's Illustrated Medical Dictionary.* Philadelphia, W.B. Saunders, 1988.

Towell, J.E. (ed.): *Acronyms, Initialisms & Abbreviations Dictionary, 1989,* 13th ed. Detroit, Gale Research, 1989.

Tuleja, T.: *Foreignisms.* New York, Macmillan, 1989.

Urdang, L.: *The Basic Book of Synonyms and Antonyms,* rev. New York, Signet, 1985.

—— (ed.): *Mosby's Medical & Nursing Dictionary.* St. Louis, C.V. Mosby, 1983.

—— (ed.): *Random House Dictionary of the English Language,* college edition. New York, Random House, 1968.

Zinsser, W.: *On Writing Well,* 3rd ed. rev. New York, Harper & Row, 1985.

Subject Index

by Linda Webster

Crossroad, 24
Crossword, 24
Cruel kindness, as oxymoron, 182
CT, 165
Cummings, Martin, 133
Cupid, 126, 174
Currently, 132
Curriculum vitae, 98
Cutting edge, as journalese and
    professionalese, 146

D.M.D., 26
Dacron, 37
Daimler company, 104
Dana, Charles A., 24
Dana Foundation, 24
Dana-Farber Cancer Institute, 24
Dangling modifiers, 44–45
Dartmouth College, 140
Dash, capitalization following in
    title, subtitle, or subhead, 22
Data, as plural, 101–2
Dates and commas, 71
Davies, Marion, 5
De rigueur, 91, 99
Deaccessioned, as bureaucratese, 6
Deacon's Masterpiece, or, The
    Wonderful One-Hoss Shay,
    140
Deafening silence, as oxymoron,
    182
Dean, Dizzy, 171
Dearth, spelling of, 91
DeBakey, Lois, 8
Deciliter, abbreviation of, 30
Decimals
    decimals that can kill, 25–26,
        32–33
    and less than one, 25, 64
    in prescriptions, 25–26, 33
    tables and, 25
Decreases, minimizes, 7
Defuse, diffuse, 111
Déjà vu, as buzz word, 146
Deliver, as medicalese, 138
Demonstrated, showed, 7
Description of investigational
    methods, 25
Descriptive and "prescriptive"
    dictionaries, 171

"Designer drug," 175
Determination, 143
Determine, 143
Dexedrine, 37
Diagnose, 139
Diagnosis, as medicalese, 139
Diagnosis, change in, 174
Dialogue, 6, 146
Dictionaries. *See also* Reference
    books
    for bad spellers, 88, 170
    descriptive and "prescriptive"
        dictionaries, 171
    directions for use of, 170
    importance of, xii
    major reference sources, 2
    purposes of, 169–70
Dictionary of American-English
    Usage, A, 52
Dictionary of Contemporary
    American Usage, 134–35
Dieresis, 78
Different from, different than,
    45–46
Differently than, 46
Diffuse, defuse, 111
Diplomat, diplomate, 112
Dis- prefix, 113
Disagreement in number of verb,
    46
Disco felon, 184
Discreet, discrete, 112
Diseases, strange, 184–85. *See also*
    names of specific diseases
Disinterested, uninterested, 112–13
Disorders, strange, 184–85
Disorganized system, as oxymoron,
    182
Displayed, listed, 11
Dissenting Opinions of Mr. Justice
    Holmes, The, 125
Dissimilar, 46
Diuresis, 139
DNA (deoxyribonucleic acid), 133
Dorland's Illustrated Medical
    Dictionary, 2
Dosage, dose, 113
Double comparatives, 64
Double helix, 133
Double meanings, 85–87

Double-spacing of manuscripts, 26
Double superlatives, 64
Down, parts of speech of, 135
Down, Down's syndrome, 27
Dragged, drug, 47
Dramatically, as medicalese, 139
Drastically, 139
Drugs and Drug Abuse, 175
Due to, 44
Duke University, 19
Dyads, dangerous, 105–28
Dyslogia, 175

E.g. (exempli gratia), 115
Each and every, 133
Early, early on, 146
Earthquakes, 183
Economy of words, 133
"Ecstasy," 175
Edit, 139
Editing. *See also* Writing
  art and science of, 7
  avoiding ambiguity in, 75
  double-spacing of manuscripts
    and, 26
  exactitude in, 7
  good judgment in, 7, 186
  knowledge in, 7
  ligatures used in, 51
  of manuscripts, 7, 26
  restraint in, 186
Education
  illiteracy of the educated and
    miseducated, 4–8
  importance of, 1, 5, 187
Education, Department of, 6
Effect, affect, 106
Effectiveness, efficacy, 113
-*efy* suffix, 94
Egregious errors in cold print,
  11–12
Either . . . or, 86
Elementary Applied Statistics, 142
Elision, 67–68
Ellipses, 73
Elsie Venner, 140
Embarrass, spelling of, 92
Employees, personnel, 148
End-point, result, 6
Endemic, 26

Energy management systems, as
    bureaucratese, 6
English. *See also* Language
  advantage of publishing in
    English, 173
  "as she is spoke," 154–62
  "death of good English," 5
  idioms in, 154
  illiteracy of the educated and
    miseducated, 4–8
  percentage of students studying,
    xii
  preservation of, 8–9
  Soviet Union students' study of,
    xii
  teutonization of, 74
  versatility of, 134–35
  versus Greek and Latin, 175
  vocabulary in everyday usage, 6
  as world language, xii–xiii, 4,
    178
Enhances, increases, 7
Enormity, immensity, 113–14
Ensurance, insurance, 47
Ensure, insure, 47
Epidemic, 26
Epistle of Paul to Timothy, 13
Epizootic, 27
Eponymous syndromes, 27–28
Eponyms, 27–28
Equal, 64
Equally as, 47
Equivocal, 6
Erlenmeyer, Emil, 92
Erlenmeyer flask, spelling of, 92
Errors
  egregious errors in cold print,
    11–12
  Freudian slips, 11–12, 15
  grammatical error, 40
  homophony and, 10–11
  in lists of references, 28
  miscomprehension, 13–14
  misquotation, 12–13
  mixed metaphors, 14
  proofreading and, 17, 85
  scrambled medical knowledge,
    15–16
  typographic errors, 15, 17, 117

Holmes, Oliver Wendell, Sr., 59,
125, 140
Holter, Norman, 16
Holter (not *halter*) monitors, 16
Hom-, homo-, 105
Home, hone, 117
Homing, 117
Homographs, 105
Homonyms, 105
Homophony, 10–11, 105
Hone, home, 117
Hopefully, 156, 157
Horace, 165
Horus, 126
Horwitz, Jerome, 19
Hospital of St. Mary of
Bethlehem, 173
Hudson, Rock, 5, 11
Hugo, Victor, 40
Human immunodeficiency virus
(HIV), 19
Humans, differentiation from
animals, 3
Hung, hanged, 117
Hydrochloride, abbreviation of, 24
Hygeia, 21
Hypersensitivity, 77
Hyphenation
adverbs modifying adjectives,
74
chemical substances as
modifiers, 74–75
compound verbs, 75–76
cross words, 24
of foreign phrases, 76, 131
general rules concerning, 73–74
hyphens as clarifiers, 75
in vitro, in vivo, 76
medical conditions and entities,
77
non-, co-, -less, and other affixes,
77–78
nouns combined with
adjectives, 78
nouns linked with nouns, 78
in personal names, 28
prefixes and proper nouns,
78–79
re- words, 79
spelled-out words and numerals,
79

of *state of the art,* 153
in titles, 28–29
unhealthful hyphens, 79–80
word processor and, 80
year-long, 80
Hypotension, 77
Hysteric, hysterical, 38

I.e. (id est), 115
I.V., as abbreviation, 23
I, we, 48
-ic, -ical words, 37–38
-ics words, plurals of, 100
Idioms, in spoken English, 154
If, as, and when, 133
If, whether, 49
-ify suffix, 94
Il- prefix, 95, 177
Ileum, ileus, 117
Illegal, 177
Illegible, 177
Illiteracy of the educated and
miseducated, 4–8
Illiteracy, statistics on, 6
Im- prefix, 95, 177
Imaging, 32
Immature, 177
Immensity, enormity, 113–14
Immoral, 177
Impact, as jargon, 6, 145
Imply, infer, 117–18
Important, 152
Impossible, 177
Impressive, 152
Improvise, 177
Imuran, 19
In, into, 49
In aeternum, spelling of, 93
In another vein, 85, 86
In any case, 86
In concert, in consort, 91
In invidiam, spelling of, 93
In lieu of, in light of, 13–14
In memoriam, spelling of, 93
In order to, 130
In perpetuum, spelling of, 93
In regard to, 45
In terms of, 6
In testimonium, spelling of, 93

Like (as preposition, not conjunction), 159
Like, such as, 87
-like suffix, 79
Likewise, 77
Lindberg, Donald A. B., x, 8
Lingua franca, 178
Linnaeus, 38
Linné, Carl von, 38
Lipmann, Fritz A., 94, 133
Liquefy, spelling of, 94
List of Journals Indexed in Index Medicus (JIM), 36
Listed, displayed, 11
Listening, 7
Lists of references. *See* Reference lists
Liter, abbreviation of, 30
Liter, equivalent measures of, 30
Literally, figuratively, 119–20
Livid, 152
Lobotomy, 12
Locum tenens, plural of, 103
Lodgment, 89
Logic, logical, 38
Logodaedaly, 167
Logotype, 30
Loma Prieta earthquake, 183
-long suffix, 80
Lord of all being! throned afar, 140
Lou Gehrig's disease, Lugerics disease, 16
Louis XIV, 9
Love's Cure, 108
Lucan, 2
Lugerics disease, Lou Gehrig's disease, 16
Lully, Jean Baptiste, 9
Lupus erythematosus, spelling of, 94–95
-ly words, 74, 120

McGill University, 181
Macleod, John, 173
Main, 152
Mainly, 156
Major, 152
Malabsorption, spelling of, 95
Malapropisms, 154–55
Malcolm X, 72

Male and female, as medicalese, 140–41
Malik, Yakov, 185
Malorthographitis, 89
Man, as generic pronoun, 12
Manner, manor, 10
Manor, manner, 10
Manual of Style (AMA), 37
Manuals
    instruction, 6
    users', 170
Manuscripts
    abbreviations in, 163–65
    block form of paragraphing in, 29
    double-spacing of, 26
    justified lines in, 29
    unjustified right margins in, 29
Many, multiple, 6
MAO, 165
Markedly, 139
Marshal, martial, 10
Marti-Ibañez, Felix, 30
Martial, marshal, 10
Martyr by accident, 7
Marx, Harpo, 126
Masonite, 37
Masterful, masterly, 120
Maximal, 65
Maximize, 64, 65, 145
MD, M.D., 81, 82, 167
Me, myself, 160–61
Mean, median, average, 120
Meanhim syndrome, 158
Meanings, double, 85–87
Measure, 143
Measurement, 143
Medium
    as catchall, 7
    plural of, 101–2
Median, mean, average, 120
Medical conditions and entities, hyphenation of, 77
Medical Essays, 140
Medical knowledge, scrambled, 15–16
Medical Literature Analysis and Retrieval System. *See* MEDLARS

Medicalese. *See also* Jargon; Journalese; Professionalese
examples of, 137–44
Medicament, medication, medicine, 121
Medication, medicine, medicament, 121
Medicine, medication, medicament, 121
MEDLARS, 163, 166
MEDLINE, 34, 166
Men and women, 141
Mercalli, Giuseppe, 183
Mercedes-Benz, 103–4
Merck Index, 34–35, 93
Merck Manual, 34, 138
Mercury, 20–21
Merriam-Webster Inc., xiv, 2, 181
Merthiolate, 37
MeSH, 166
Metaphors. *See* Mixed metaphors
Method, 141
Methodology, as medicalese, 139–40
Methods, description of, 25
Mice, nude, 180
Michigan Cancer Foundation, 19
Mickey mouse, as buzz word, 146
Micron, plural of, 103
Microorganisms. *See* Bacteria
Midchest, 77
Military intelligence, as oxymoron, 182
Militate, mitigate, 121
Milk of magnesia, 37
Millennium, spelling of, 95
Miller-Abbott tube, 28
Milliliter, abbreviation of, 30
Milton, John, 182
Minimize, minimum, 64–65
Minimizes, decreases, 7
Minimum, minimize, 64–65
Minister, administer, 62
Minor breakthrough, as bureaucratese, 7
Minuscule, spelling of, 95
Mish, Frederick C., xiv, 181
Misquotation, 12–13
Miss Thistlebottom's Hobgoblins, xi

Misspelled words, 88–99
Mistakes. *See* Errors
Mitchell, Richard, 42
Mitigate, militate, 121
"Mixaphors," 14
Mixed metaphors, 14
Mnemonic, 106
Mnemonic aids, 166
Mnemosyne, 106
Modality, as medicalese, 141
Mode, 141
Modern American Usage, 38, 48, 59
Modern English Usage, 52
Modifiers. *See also* Adjectives; Adverbs
agglomeration of, 135–36
chemical substances as modifiers, 74–75
dangling modifiers, 44–45
nouns as, 134–36
Mokusatsu, 183–84
"Money as root of all evil," 13
Month-long, 80
Moral turpitude, 40
Morbidity, mortality, 30
Morbidity, mortality rates, 30
More important(ly), 45, 158
Morphine, 18
Mortality, morbidity, 30
Mortality, morbidity rates, 30
Most as superlative, 64
Mourning Bride, 12
Moynihan, Daniel P., 185
MRI, 32
Mucus, mucous, 95–96
Multifactoral, multifactorial, 121
Multiple, many, 6
Muses, 106
"Music has charms," 12
Myself, me, 160–61
Mythology, 20–21, 106, 126, 174

Nagasaki, 184
NAILS, 166–67
Naloxone, 18
Names. *See* Proper nouns
Natatory, 172
National Air and Space Museum, 35

National Armed Forces Museum
Advisory Board, 35
National Cancer Institute, 19
National Collection of Fine Arts,
35
National Formulary names, 34
National Gallery of Art, 35
National Library of Medicine
(NLM), 8, 133, 163, 166
National Museum of Design, 35
National Museum of History and
Technology, 35
National Museum of Natural
History, 35
National Portrait Gallery, 35
National Zoological Park, 35
Native Tongues, 183
Nausea, 122
Nauseated, nauseous, 121–22
Necropsy, 139
Needless to say, 152
Neither . . . nor, verb form with,
55–56
Nembutal, 37
Neonates, 140
Neonatology, 19
Nephroblastoma, 27
Neubauer-Fischer test, 28
New York Times, 12, 70, 169
*New York Times Winners and
Sinners*, 61, 116
Newborns, 140
Newton, Sir Isaac, 2
NF (National Formulary) names,
34
Nicholson, Margaret, 52
NLM. *See* National Library of
Medicine (NLM)
NMRI, 32
Nobel prize, 173
Non- prefix, hyphenation of, 77
None, verb form with, 55
Nonnegotiable, 77
Nonproprietary and proprietary
names, 33–35
Nonsense, 77
Nor- prefix, 179
Normal, abnormal, as medicalese,
137
Normal, ordinary, 122

Nostalgia, as buzz word, 146
Nouns. *See also* Proper nouns
false verbs from nouns, 139
hyphenation with nouns
combined with adjectives, 78
hyphenation with nouns linked
with nouns, 78
hyphenation with prefixes and
proper nouns, 78–79
as modifiers, 134–36
plural of proper nouns, 103–4
possessives of, 68–69
spelling of proper names, 93
use of *the late* with personal
names, 147–48
as verbs, 141
verbs from, 151
Nu gene, 180
Nuclear magnetic resonance
imaging (NMRI), 32
Nude mice, 180
Nude Mouse Secretariat (Copenhagen), 180
Number, verb form with, 55
Numbers
consistency and, 23, 31
hyphenation of spelled-out
words and numerals, 79
journalism rules for, 31
pH value, 32
at start of sentence, 164
virgule with, 38
Numerals. *See* Numbers
Nurnberg, Maxwell, 70
Nylon, 37

O.D., 33, 165
O.U., 33
Obverse, converse, inverse, reverse,
119
Obviously, clear, 152–53
Occurring, spelling of, 96
Octothorp, 180–81
œ, æ ligatures, 20, 50
Oedipus, 51
Of understood in possessives, 69
Oids, corticosteroids, 6
Old English, 54
Old Ironsides, 140
Olivier, Sir Laurence, 178

EDITH SCHWAGER

Edith Schwager, a medical editor-writer, was the Editor of the American Medical Writers Association's *AMWA Journal* for eight years. She is the author of the "Dear Edie" column in the *AMWA Journal* and a feature writer for an international drug newsmagazine. She has received virtually every national honor accorded by the AMWA, including the Swanberg and Golden Apple awards. Her workshops on English usage attract students from the United States, Canada, and Europe. She has been copy and executive editor of more than 35 books and 1,500 articles on medical, pharmaceutical, and pharmacologic topics.